CORONER

CORONER

Morton Shulman

Fitzhenry & Whiteside

Toronto Montreal Winnipeg Vancouver

ISBN 0-88902-017-5

Acknowledgement is due to *The Toronto Star* for the cartoons by Macpherson, to *The Globe and Mail* for cartoons by Reidford, to *The Toronto Sun* for cartoons by Donato and Beaton which originally appeared in *The Toronto Telegram*, to Franklin and to Fons von Woerkom for their cartoons, and to Ron Haggart for his article reprinted in chapter 22.

Design by Maher & Garbutt Ltd

Fitzhenry & Whiteside Limited
150 Lesmill Road
Don Mills, Ontario

Printed in Canada

Contents

Foreword

I am afraid that this book will provoke cries that I have blown my own horn overmuch. To those critics I can only reply that I have told it as I believe it was—I do not claim that I was any wiser than those with whom I was in conflict but rather that ours was the classic dispute between those attempting to maintain a pretty good status quo and those who believed that improvement was possible. Certainly there were no personal animosities in those battles and today I am happy to say that I meet on a friendly basis almost all of my earlier foes.

My years as Chief Coroner gave me many satisfactions but they cost me too much time away from my dear ones. This book is written so that Dianne and Jeff will know what I was doing during those busy years.

In 1970 Premier John Robarts said to me, "The biggest political mistake I made was hiring you as Chief Coroner—my second biggest was firing you."

1 *How to Become a Coroner*

When I opened my office to practise medicine in West Toronto in 1950, there was no problem in quickly building up a practice, for there had been a tremendous immigrant influx to the city and there were not enough general practitioners to handle the rush. Getting one's patients into hospital, however, was quite a different matter. Every hospital in the city had a closed list of physicians who had admission privileges and to get one's name on that list was next to impossible without influence with someone important at one of the hospitals.

This meant that the general practitioner outside hospitals could earn a very good living by seeing patients in his office and in their homes but was prevented from treating any complicated medical or surgical cases because lack of facilities forced him to refer his patients to those more fortunate physicians who had hospital appointments.

Pregnancies came into a special category. When I first went into practice I had been under the illusion that the Toronto General Hospital's Private Patients' Pavilion was open, at least as far as obstetrics was concerned, to all physicians. But I soon found that no matter when I phoned for a reservation the beds for that month were already fully booked. Finally one day I phoned to request a fictitious obstetrical booking for ten months hence but was told that all the obstetrical beds were already booked for that month.

While the Toronto General Hospital would not allow non-staff physicians into their Private Patients' Pavilion, it did maintain a somewhat lower-class establishment, the Burnside, which welcomed all physicians. Since the accommodation was rather drab and uncomfortable this effectively limited outside doctors' obstetrical practice to the less affluent residents of the city.

My own office was only a few blocks from St. Joseph's Hospital, and I found that the Sister Superior was willing to allow me the very occasional obstetrical bed provided that the patient was Roman Catholic and the reservation was made at least seven months in advance. This situation did not last for long, however. One day I was called in to see the Sister Superior, who greeted me with a large smile.

"All doctors who deliver patients in this hospital should be on staff, so I wondered if you would mind filling out a staff application form—that is if you would like to be on our staff."

I was pleased and hurried to fill out the form. Three days later I was informed that my application had been refused and therefore they were very sorry but I could not deliver any more patients at St. Joseph's Hospital.

By accepting overflow and night calls from other doctors and from the Academy of Medicine, I rapidly built up a large practice, though it demanded sixteen-hour days and constant running. But I was becoming more and more frustrated by being unable to treat anything more complicated than the 'flu because of the closed-door policy of all the general hospitals in Toronto. This problem began to be resolved one night at 3:00 a.m. when I received an urgent phone call to come to see a Mr. Jack Barnet who lived just around the corner from my combined office and home on Roncesvalles Avenue.

Jack Barnet was then thirty-eight years old, an aggressive ward politician who had carved a small empire out for himself in the downtown St. Patrick's riding. He had parlayed two rooming houses into a stake with which he had purchased the Turf Club Hotel, a flourishing beer parlour right across the street from the Toronto General Hospital. He had developed his connections from this little hotel into a political machine which had been successful in getting elected both a federal member of parliament and a provincial member. Barnet was riding very high and he took great pride in pointing out that he had come from the slums of Pembroke Street but now lunched at Toronto's prestigious Albany Club with the likes of the Speaker of the House of Commons (and later Governor General) Roland Michener.

Barnet was very impressed with my coming to see him in the wee hours and I soon became the family doctor. As Jack had recently married his long-time sweetheart Mary and she was now pregnant, he asked me to make a reservation for her delivery at Toronto General Hospital's Private Patients' Pavilion.

I explained my position as a non-staff-physician to Jack Barnet and suggested that he call one of the obstetricians on the staff at the General. His reaction was typical: "Those dirty bastards, we'll show them. I'll make you a coroner."

A coroner—entré to the hospitals, $10.00 a call and always paid, the excitement of interesting cases and the challenge of investigations! My head pounded with the vision.

The coroner's office for generations had been a closed shop to which only very lofty WASP members of the establishment were admitted. Some years before one Roman Catholic, a Dr. O'Hara and one Jew, Dr. L. J. Breslin had been appointed coroners in order to minimize complaints from minorities, but their appointments were made on condition that they agreed not to go on any calls and through their lifetime neither received a coroner call. The coroner's office was used as a dumping ground for cases embarrassing either to the government or the medical profession. Such cases were speedily and efficiently disposed of without any embarrassment to any influential person and yet smoothly enough that there had never been a public complaint.

Barnet immediately began his campaign to have me appointed. I joined the Progressive Conservative party, went to political meetings, lunched with MP Roly Michener and MPP Ted Reay at the Albany and Granite clubs and even went to see Chief Coroner Smirle Lawson to ensure his benevolent neutrality. (Although Dr. Lawson had nothing to do with the appointment of coroners, if someone were appointed of whom he did not approve he would assign them to the outskirts of the city where they received practically no calls.)

Alas, all was in vain. Jack Barnet had been having difficulties with his business and had begun to slip badly. Soon he was taking sleeping pills to put himself to sleep at night and dexedrine to get himself going in the morning. On this regimen he went downhill rapidly, lost his grip on both his business and his politics and literally tired of living. He died in 1951 at the age of thirty-nine.

The idea of a coronership still obsessed me and so I approached Mr. W. J. Stewart, the former MPP for West Toronto, to seek his help. Bill Stewart had had a unique career; he had been Toronto's depression mayor, had distinguished himself in the Ontario legislature and had been appointed Speaker of the House and then had been forced out by Premier George Drew. In 1951 he was working actively to regain his seat as a member of the provincial legislature which he had lost in the previous election to the CCF (now the NDP). I had a large practice in Mr. Stewart's riding of Parkdale and I took time to visit each of my patients to solicit support for Bill Stewart. In early 1952 he won the seat by an overwhelming majority. Two months later I received my appointment as a city coroner.

The day the appointment came through I received a phone call from a local politician who informed me that the customary fee for a coronership was $2,000. I scraped the cash together and went to Mr. Stewart's office. I began: "Mr. Stewart, I want to reimburse you for your expenses in going to all this trouble."

"Great, come in and sit down. The cost will be two car tickets, one down and one back. Morton, I have been in politics all my life and I have never accepted a penny even for my campaign expenses. I would not want to begin at this late date. All I want from you is your friendship and support."

Bill Stewart and I remained close friends until his death in 1970. He was a man of great integrity and honesty who was shabbily treated by his party after his final defeat at the polls.

Now I made a second visit to Smirle Lawson. Dr. Lawson was a living legend, a huge, powerful man who was renowned for his unique direct methods. He was the only student in the history of the University of Toronto to ever get 100 in surgery and this feat was achieved when the professor of surgery wagered with him that he would not score six touchdowns at the next game with Queens. For many years there hung at the coroner's office a picture of

Smirle Lawson charging across the goal line with four opposing players being dragged behind.

Dr. Lawson believed in loyalty and kindness but this loyalty had lead the coroner's office down a strange path. He issued only three instructions to me upon assuming my duties: "(1) Look after the poor widows — the rich can look after themselves. (2) When you see an eighty-year-old man lying dead in bed, don't search under the bed for a gun. (3) Don't cause any trouble for the government and especially not for the medical profession. If a doctor does something wrong take him in the back room and give him hell, but don't let the public or the press learn about it."

His welcome to me that first day was nerve-racking. He took me to the Crown Attorney's office and insisted on introducing me to everyone as "Morton Shulman, my new coroner—he's a Jew, isn't that amazing?" The embarrassed crown attorneys wished me well and hurried away. Smirle Lawson was certainly not anti-semitic. He just believed that every person and every group had their fixed place on this earth and he found it amazing that a Jewish doctor could be appointed to this post.

2 The Coroner at Work

Most people misunderstand the role of the coroner, confusing him with the pathologist; so when I became a coroner I was continually being asked how I could stand cutting up dead bodies. Actually coroners never do post-mortems and the coroner's role largely consists of examining the circumstances of the death. If there is some question about the cause of death the coroner will order a pathologist to do an autopsy.

My typical day as a coroner would begin at 8:00 A.M. with a call from the Chief Coroner's office, giving the bare details of a death at a local hospital—name, address and age of the deceased plus the location in the hospital. I would breakfast and then go to the hospital where I would examine the medical records of the deceased. Ninety per cent of these cases were elderly patients who had died without previous medical care and I would merely sign the death certificate and make out my report. In those few cases where death was the result of violence I would order the body sent to the morgue for an autopsy.

The morgue itself on Lombard Street also contained the Chief Coroner's office and a courtroom for inquests. It was, and is, a stark, mid-nineteenth century, two-storey building with a courtroom on the top floor and the offices and the storage facilities for dead bodies in the rudimentary post-mortem room on the main floor. The proximity of the various quarters resulted in a constant unpleasant odour of death, particularly in the courtroom which was immediately above the autopsy room. There were no amenities and the furniture consisted of three desks and half a dozen hardback chairs. Visitors to the morgue never tarried. I made repeated pleas to City Council for money to modernize the building but this was never forthcoming and I well recall that a request to City Council for $50 to buy drapes for the room in which relatives would identify their dead was refused.

Perhaps once or twice a day I would receive a call when someone had died in his home or in a public place, for instance in a car accident. These cases required immediate attention and I would then leave everything else and would hurry to the scene where I would be met by a police officer. Many of these cases required a post-mortem.

After I received the results of the post-mortem from the pathologist (and this took anywhere from a few hours to several weeks depending on how much technical investigation was required), I would decide whether an inquest was called for. In a few types of death inquests were mandatory, for example, the death of a prisoner in a jail or an inmate in a mental institution, but usually the decision was up to the coroner. In those days inquests were held mainly when the family was complaining, or when there had been considerable publicity surrounding the death, and their purpose was, as Smirle Lawson put it, "to clear the air."

Inquests followed less than 1 percent of the deaths but resulted in 99 percent of the publicity a coroner received. In his investigations a coroner played the parts of both doctor and detective, and in his inquests he acted the roles of investigating attorney and judge. An inquest is a courtroom investigation presided over by the coroner, sometimes assisted by a crown attorney, with a jury of five men or women hearing sworn evidence from all the witnesses who had information about the death. After all the witnesses had testified the coroner would sum up the evidence for the jury, give them his recommendations to prevent similar deaths and ask them to retire and bring in a verdict. The jury rarely failed to echo the coroner's summary and recommendations.

Up until 1961 the coroner had one other duty and this was to examine rape victims for sperm and signs of violence. Invariably these calls came from the police in the small hours and I would go to the emergency ward of one of the downtown hospitals where I would find a weeping woman or child in hysteria. This job of the coroner had never been spelled out in law but had been instituted by Dr. Smirle Lawson at the request of the police and the hospitals. When Dr. Beatty Cotnam became supervising coroner he ordered this practice stopped and most of us were greatly relieved, although the police complained bitterly.

Overall the job was an exciting one and soon I was running on up to ten calls a week investigating murders, suicides and other assorted mayhem. I found the work fascinating, but I soon learned there were certain boundaries that could not be crossed.

Two months after receiving my appointment I was called to investigate a case at St. Michael's Hospital in which in my opinion death had resulted from negligence on the part of a physician. I ordered a post-mortem and returned to my office. Half an hour later Smirle Lawson called and ordered me to return at once to St. Michael's Hospital where he said he would meet me in the Sister Superior's office. When I arrived at the hospital Dr. Lawson informed me that he was taking over the case and that I must cancel the post-mortem. There seemed little choice, and I did what I was told. He then instructed me to apologize to the Sister Superior. With tail very much between my legs I returned to my office, resolved never to go through such a humiliating experience again.

Once this lesson had been taught Dr. Lawson returned to his exuberant friendly self. He was unfailingly kind to me, generous with his advice and when I made the inevitable learning blunders he always backed me up. Learning proper behaviour was one of the serious problems in coroners' work at that time. There was no course or organized teaching of any type and new coroners depended entirely on Edward Armour, the long-time coroner's clerk. Eddy Armour was a little gnome of a man, bald, about five feet tall, with sharp restless eyes that didn't miss a thing. He had worked at the Coroner's Office for close to thirty years and had reached the point where he handled Dr. Lawson's correspondence, with the Chief Coroner coming into the office at very infrequent intervals. Eddy Armour even signed Dr. Lawson's letters, a hazardous practice, as later events proved.

Each coroner's report had to be signed by the coroner and then the signature had to be witnessed by a commissioner for oaths. Dr. Lawson told me that Eddy Armour was the commissioner who should witness my signature. At the end of my first month I had done ten cases and when I brought the forms down to the office Eddy informed me: "That will be $5 — 50 cents a signature." I paid. The next month I had twenty cases. When he found I caused no difficulty I soon went up to my average of fifty cases a month which represented a very substantial part of my income.

One thing a coroner should be able to tell is whether his client is dead or alive. Early in my career as assistant coroner I was sent on two cases which I shall never forget. Both took place in 1954, the first one at St. Joseph's Hospital where a physician had not pronounced the patient dead but the nun on duty had decided that the patient had expired and called the coroner's office. When I arrived on the floor the nurse on duty directed me to the proper room, but when I entered to examine the body a very live gentleman sitting in the bed demanded to know what was my business with him. "They told me you were dead," I blurted, and he roared back at me, "You are all crazy, get me my clothes, I'm going home." I made a hasty retreat and informed the nurse and sister that their body was very much alive. I recall that they seemed quite put out with both me and the patient. The nurse urged me to wait as she was certain the man was almost, if not quite, dead but I left hastily. Coroners were paid by the call and I remember asking Smirle Lawson if I could charge for a call when the patient had recovered. He said, "Mileage only, my boy!"

The second case was even more disconcerting. I received a call that someone had died on the operating table at the Sick Children's Hospital and when I arrived I was told that the body was still on the table in the operating room. When I entered the room I approached the operating table on which lay a body covered with a sheet. To my horror as I reached the table the body slowly began to sit up. I gave a horrified shriek and ran from the room to accompanying gales of laughter from the assembled interns. Shortly before my arrival the body had been removed to the hospital morgue and its place taken by one of the interns. I thought that it showed an odd sense of humour.

Much later, in 1966, when I was Chief Coroner, we had a more distressing experience at the morgue, when one of the bodies came to life shortly before an autopsy was to begin. A Toronto coroner had been called to an apartment to examine the body of a fifty-seven-year-old woman, apparently dead from an overdose of drugs. Police had been called by relatives who were concerned about the woman's health and had gone to see her. When the officers found the woman lying in the bathroom in her pyjamas they notified the coroner.

The coroner in charge of the case later explained, "The patient was certainly cold, there was no respiration noticeable at the time and no apparent pulse. I examined her twice. She was in a warm room but was cold as death and had the typical pallor. I gave her a thorough examination and re-checked." The doctor made out a death certificate and ordered the body taken to the morgue for an autopsy to determine the cause of death. At the morgue the ambulance men left the body strapped on a stretcher while they went to find an empty locker to put it in.

As the nineteen-year-old ambulance driver put it, "I went back into the autopsy room to get her and suddenly she moved. I raced out the door yelling 'She's alive!' I admit I was frightened. After all, that does not happen every day."

The "body" was transferred to hospital and the coroner was suspended.

In the mid-fifties the routine varied little. I did as many calls as each of the other five active city coroners but if the case were one in which the press showed an interest or which might prove embarrassing to the government, a few days before the inquest I would receive a phone call from Smirle Lawson.

"I am very interested in this particular case, Morton, do you mind if I take over the inquest? I will tell Eddy to give you another case instead."

I had no choice and always replied, "Yes, Sir."

The inquests themselves were not models of justice. The jurors were chosen from a small list of friends which was maintained by Smirle's court constable, a Sergeant Quackenbush, who was closely attuned to Smirle's desires. When the jury retired Quackenbush would go with them and would help them write the verdict, which invariably coincided with Smirle's wishes — or in his absence with what Quackenbush thought Smirle would have wished. Quackenbush finally retired in 1960.

Gradually as the years passed Smirle began to trust me more and this, associated with his increasing age, led him to allow me to handle more important cases. By 1960 he had almost completely given up conducting inquests and I was handling all the sensitive investigations for the coroner's office.

3 *How to Become Chief Coroner*

"Smirle Lawson has accused you of forging his signature!"

As Dr. Lawson came toward the end of his career, the Attorney General's department became anxious about the situation at the Coroner's Office. Dr. Lawson had held the two positions of Chief Coroner for Toronto and Supervising Coroner for Ontario for over twenty years and the entire coroner system was tightly under his control. The Attorney General's department felt that procedures had become lax and out of date, and there was open speculation in the department that Smirle was becoming senile. For some time now he had made a habit of walking about with his shoelaces undone, and there were other and more embarrassing incidents of absent-mindedness.

For over two years from 1959 the Attorney General's department sought, without success, Dr. Lawson's resignation. The suggestion was even made to a *Globe and Mail* reporter, Harold Greer, that there was a good story in the Coroner's Office. He wrote a series of articles under the general heading *Are Coroners Necessary?* and listed a number of weaknesses in the system. I did my duty to Dr. Lawson by writing, at his request, a letter to the *Globe* editor stoutly defending the coroner system and Dr. Lawson's administration.

The Attorney General's department then used Greer's series as reason to set up a commission to look into the workings of the Coroner's Office. The commission, consisting of the Assistant

Deputy Attorney General, Eric Silk (who later became head of the Ontario Provincial Police), Dr. H. Ward Smith, head of the Crime Laboratory, and Dr. David Gemmell, a coroner from Stratford who had ambitions to replace Smirle Lawson. They made various recommendations, including more extensive supervision and guidance from the Supervising Coroner's Office, but Dr. Lawson would not budge. Now feeling the pressure, Dr. Lawson marched down to the office of the Attorney General to threaten that if he were fired all his coroners would quit with him. He suggested/ordered that we all accompany him, but of the eight city coroners only Fred Tickett and I appeared on this kamikaze mission, and Fred whispered to me as we entered the office, "You wouldn't really quit, would you? I certainly won't."

In fact there was little likelihood of Dr. Lawson being fired because the political repercussions would have been too threatening if he had decided to tell his stories of past scandals. Smirle Lawson was not sure of this however, and in an effort to stave off the inevitable he kept promising that he would retire "next year." Finally, one evening in September 1961 Dr. Lawson phoned me, said he had decided to retire in 1962 when he would have completed twenty-five years of service, and asked me to type out and bring over his resignation. He went on to say that he wanted me to succeed him.

With my wife I went to the address he gave me in North Toronto where I found a party in progress. Dr. Lawson took me out to a balcony and started to sign the resignation. Fortunately for my future I requested that he call out one of his friends to read the resignation with him, and to act as a witness. The next morning I sent the resignation to Mr. Kelso Roberts, the Attorney General.

Two weeks later I was at a Conservative meeting when my friend Bill Stewart came up to me and said, "Have you heard the latest about Smirle? He has accused Eric Silk of forging his signature on a resignation with the help of Eddy Armour."

I was appalled and proceeded to make what came close to being a fatal error. I phoned Dr. Lawson's home, was told that he was ill and spoke to Mrs. Lawson. "Eric Silk didn't forge Dr. Lawson's signature, he signed that resignation in my presence." Mrs. Lawson angrily replied, "You knew Smirle had had a lot to drink that night, you shouldn't have sent it in." She hung up.

The next day I learned to my horror that Dr. Lawson had now accused me of forging the resignation and that he had denied ever seeing it. He withdrew his accusation against Eric Silk. He, his wife and a handwriting expert now made an appointment to see the Attorney General, and I was frantic. I began to search for the friend of Dr. Lawson who had witnessed the signing of his resignation. I knew that his name was Al Simpson and that he ran a furniture store somewhere near Holland Marsh, but I did not know the address or phone number. I drove up to Holland Marsh, went to the provincial police and asked if they knew where I could locate him. His store was a hundred yards from the police station.

I walked into Al Simpson's store and came right to the point, "Mr. Simpson, I am in serious trouble. Smirle Lawson denies ever signing that resignation and claims I forged his signature. Will you help me?" To my great relief Al Simpson replied, "Of course he signed it, I read it to him and saw him sign it! I will give you an affidavit to that effect." I drove back to Toronto with the affidavit witnessed by a police officer and the next morning I took it to the Attorney General. Later, when Smirle and Mrs. Lawson had their appointment with Mr. Roberts, the Attorney General said to Dr. Lawson, "Okay, Smirle, let's get down to brass tacks. I gather you don't want to quit in January. When will you quit?" Dr. Lawson replied, "I want six months, I'll quit in June." The two men shook hands on the deal.

Mrs. Lawson began to protest. "But I have a certificate here from a handwriting expert saying that this is not Smirle's signature." Dr. Lawson grabbed it from her and threw it in the wastebasket, gave Mr. Roberts a wink and said, "Let's forget that."

For the ensuing seven months until Dr. Lawson's resignation went into effect I expected trouble but my fears were groundless. Dr. Lawson had returned to his former courteous self on the few occasions on which I saw him and I continued to do the same amount of work as before.

I did hear, however, that behind the scenes the Lawsons were working hard to ensure the appointment of Dr. Jack Lovering as Chief Coroner. A tremendous struggle now developed, as there were two other candidates for this position.

Jack Lovering, fortyish and bright, had been a coroner for some fifteen years. He now had Dr. Lawson's all-out support but he made no real effort on his own behalf to get the position. He would have accepted it gratefully but was busily occupied with his medical practice and his duties as medical director of a large oil company. Gerald Blanchet was a young coroner who actively set out to get the job by lining up the support of as many medical groups as possible. Alison Noble was a coroner from a Toronto suburb who had not worked in the city proper up to that time and who received his support from his local MPP. I was very ambitious and anxious to get the post and sought the support of Kelso Roberts, the Attorney General.

In 1961 the Premier of Ontario, Leslie Frost, had decided to retire and a Progressive Conservative party convention had been called for the end of October to choose a new leader. There were seven candidates, one of whom was the relatively unknown Minister of Education, John Robarts.

The Attorney General had summoned me to his office and said, "I would like your support for my bid for the leadership. I know you want to be Chief Coroner, and I will see that you are appointed. If I succeed in my bid I will be premier and if I don't I will still be Attorney General. Could you deliver the eighteen votes from Parkdale riding?"

I was by now the president of the Parkdale riding Progressive Conservative Association and most of the members of the executive were friends of mine. A meeting was called that week and delegates were named for the convention which was to be held the following month. Everyone agreed to support Kelso Roberts. What we didn't know was that Arthur Maloney, who was our local federal member of Parliament, had promised John Robarts that he would deliver the same eighteen votes to him. A sharp struggle now ensued within the riding association but as the delegates had already been named there was little Mr. Maloney could do and ultimately sixteen of the votes were cast at the convention for Mr. Roberts.

Kelso Roberts headed the polls on the first ballot but as one after another of the seven other candidates were eliminated John Robarts drew ahead. When on the final ballot Bob Macaulay threw his support to Mr. Robarts it was all over.

With John Robarts' victory Kelso Roberts' long political career was over; he remained for a few more months as Attorney General but with lessening power. When I approached him for his support for the job of Chief Coroner he explained the situation frankly, "I am barely holding on to my own job and have no way to get you the appointment I promised you. Look elsewhere — you have no future here."

Shortly afterwards I read in the press that on the retirement of Dr. Smirle Lawson, his post of Supervising Coroner of Ontario was to be filled by Dr. Beatty Cotnam of Pembroke and the lower but more important post of Chief Coroner of Metro Toronto was to be left vacant. I then decided to enter active politics and run for office.

I was still in control of the Parkdale Progressive Conservative Association. My old friend Bill Stewart had been the Conservative candidate in the previous provincial election and had been defeated by the Liberal Jim Trotter who now appeared unbeatable. The riding was still represented federally by Conservative Arthur Maloney so federal politics were out. I decided to run against Trotter but I knew I needed a good issue in order to have any chance of winning.

During the fifties there had been increasing controversy over the then revolutionary new idea of medicare, culminating in its introduction by the CCF government in Saskatchewan and the subsequent strike by the doctors of that province. The Tories of Ontario had no intention of seeking similar troubles and had reassured the medical profession of their province that they had nothing to fear. On the other hand, I had seen too many examples in my own practice of families postponing essential medical treatment because they could not afford the expense. I felt that the time had come to bring medicare to Ontario and I was anxious to test my ideas at the polls.

In December 1962 I convened a meeting of the members of the executive of the Parkdale Progressive Conservative Association and told them that I was willing to run against Trotter but only on condition that they endorsed my platform which would be the introduction of a system of prepaid medical care run by the government. They were hungry for a victory and voted unanimously to support me. We decided to call a nominating convention for the following month.

I now had the support of my local organization but had no idea what the reaction would be from party headquarters. Obviously my task at the polls would become an impossible one if I were to be disowned by John Robarts. On January 5, 1963, I wrote the Premier telling him that I was seeking the Parkdale nomination, was supported by the entire executive and intended to run on a platform of medicare. I asked him neither to support nor disown me but to let the people decide, for as I put it to him, "If I am defeated you will have lost nothing, for the seat appears solidly Liberal, and on the other hand, if I am elected I believe that you should then give serious consideration to the introduction of a government medicare scheme."

Robarts was appalled and moved quickly to neutralize this potential embarrassment. One week later I received a phone call from one Dalton Bales, whose name I had never heard before but who was to play an important part in my future. Bales introduced himself as speaking for the Premier and invited me to attend a meeting the following day in the office of Hugh Latimer, the secretary of the provincial Progressive Conservative pary.

The next day I was warmly greeted by these two behind-the-scenes operators who told me that the Conservative party would be happy to have me as an MPP but that it seemed a terrible waste to lose my proven talents in the coroners' field. Would I instead consider taking the post of Chief Coroner of Metropolitan Toronto? I fell over myself saying "Yes," and then Latimer said, "Oh there's one thing we want you to do first. We have a potential candidate for Parkdale riding, a fine young Polish lawyer by the name of Casimir Bielski. We would like him to get the nomination and would like your help, if, of course, you think after meeting him that he would make a good candidate and MPP." I said that of course I would meet him and Dalton Bales then added, "Great—he is in the next room so let us call him in so that you two can get acquainted."

At this point I would have endorsed Godzilla and it took me all of thirty seconds to tell Latimer and Bales that I was sure that Cas

Bielski would make an excellent candidate. However, I warned them that if I endorsed Bielski, then Arthur Maloney, who was still the Federal Member, would automatically oppose him because he was still annoyed with me over the Robarts-Roberts fiasco. Dalton Bales replied, "Well surely, Dr. Shulman, if you are going to handle the major problems of the Coroner's Office, you should be able to handle a simple nominating convention." I assured him that I would manage it somehow, although I felt anything but confident.

The following week the Parkdale PC's held their monthly executive meeting and I took Bielski with me while I made my pitch. Arthur Maloney sat unsmiling in the first row. I spoke long and persuasively, explaining why I was not running and urging these long-time WASP residents of Parkdale to accept an ethnic candidate in view of the increasing percentage of non-WASP residents of Parkdale. When I sat down I felt that I had not persuaded them. Then Arthur Maloney rose and I thought: "There it goes—I blew it." But to my utter amazement Maloney supported me, ending up, "I have learned that Morton Shulman's political judgment is excellent. If he is nominating Cas Bielski I wish to have the privilege of seconding him." Bielski won the nomination unanimously.

It was not until a year later that I learned the background to this strange political story. Maloney had wanted to nominate Bielski but had the same fears that I had, namely that if he proposed I would oppose. So he had carefully arranged that I would bring Bielski to Parkdale. It was all in vain, for Jimmy Trotter clobbered Bielski in the election the following year.

But not entirely in vain. In March 1963, on the recommendation of the new Attorney General, Fred Cass, I was appointed Chief Coroner of Metropolitan Toronto.

4 *Into Battle*

My four years as Chief Coroner were exciting ones but were marred from the very beginning by a running battle with various government officials, particularly the senior officials in the department of the Attorney General.

My troubles had begun before my appointment was confirmed. There had been a tragic accident in Toronto's east-west subway which was then under construction. A tunnel had collapsed killing several men and I had ordered an inquest. Deputy Attorney General William Common assigned an assistant to act as the Crown Attorney and a few days before the inquest the assistant phoned me to inform me that he had selected five citizens to be on the jury; one was a town planner, one was an official of the labourers' unions, and one was a representative of the construction industry. I was flabbergasted and told the representative of the Crown Attorney that there was no way he could choose the jury and that this jury, like all others, would be chosen by lot. He was furious and ordered me to comply and when I refused he said that if I did not cooperate one of us would have to withdraw from the case. I informed him that I had already issued my warrant for the inquest and whether or not he was present was of no consequence to me.

The next day the furious assistant threw in the towel and the inquest proceeded in the normal way. He bore no hard feelings and we subsequently became friends. Alas, my battles with more senior officials in the Attorney General's department were not as successful.

Four weeks after my appointment as Chief Coroner thirty-year-old Louis Pisecny drowned after falling out of a small boat in Toronto Bay. The boat had carried no life jackets and I was shocked to read in the press that very same day that the federal Department of Transport was about to change its regulations to remove the requirement that small boats carry life jackets.

I have always believed that the main, sometimes the sole, purpose of an inquest is to present recommendations which will prevent similar deaths in the future. It appeared obvious to me that Pisecny's death could be used to save other lives by pointing out to the public the need to have life jackets in small boats. It may have appeared obvious but various civil servants did not agree with me.

The inquest convened on May 9 and the key witness was one Thomas Appleton, a Small Boats Officer with the Marine Regulations Board of the federal Department of Transport. I asked Appleton what was the reasoning behind the proposed new regulations but he flatly refused to give his opinion, saying that he was only responsible for enforcing regulations and couldn't discuss them. Under the circumstances I did not think that the jury could come to a fair conclusion and so I adjourned the inquest to May 29 to allow time to subpoena a more senior member of the department who would be able and qualified to advise the jury.

The roof now quickly proceeded to fall in. The Deputy Minister of Transport in Ottawa called his friend Dr. Christie, the Assistant Deputy Minister of Justice in Ottawa, asking Christie to use his influence to stop that pesky coroner in Toronto from embarrassing the department. Christie now called Bill Common, the Deputy Attorney General of Ontario, and Common in turn called Dr. Beatty Cotnam, the Supervising Coroner of Ontario. Dr. Cotnam wrote me to tell me that "there has been considerable discussion from various government departments in Ottawa concerning the conduct of the above inquest." He asked for an explanation which I supplied.

Bill Common now wrote a letter to Henry Bull, the Crown Attorney of York County, saying, "This is not a case for an expert witness; moreover the opinion of civil servants in relation to legislative policy of their government should not under any circumstances be entertained or even requested. I am confident that you will make it perfectly clear to Dr. Shulman that under no circumstances must he explore this aspect of the matter."

Henry Bull complied with his boss's order and wrote me: "There seems to be no purpose to be served in bringing the witness from Ottawa, as he would have no relevant evidence to give. However, I have said that, unless the subpoena is withdrawn, it will be necessary for him to attend at the resumed hearing although objection will be taken to any opinion evidence that might be called for. May I have your advice that the subpoena has been withdrawn and the witness need not attend for any purpose."

I had no idea what I should do—I certainly had little stomach for a battle with the Crown Attorney, the Deputy Attorney General, the Supervising Coroner and the federal government. On the other hand I knew that expert evidence was essential to the proper completion of the inquest, so I decided to lay all the facts before the Attorney General, Fred Cass. That day, May 27, I wrote Mr. Cass explaining all the facts and asking for his direction. I took the letter to the Attorney General's office, handed it to his secretary and asked her to give it to him at once.

I received no reply from Fred Cass before the inquest reconvened. Captain Keith Angers, head of the Nautical Safety Division came from the Department of Transport but he was accompanied by Assistant Crown Attorney Pat Lesage, who refused to allow Captain Angers to give his opinion of the boating regulations. He said he was acting on instructions from Deputy Attorney General W.B. Common.

Despite the confusion the jury recommended that the government require all small boats to carry life jackets.

The next day the Toronto *Telegram* editorialized on the foolishness of the federal-provincial legalisms in their "attempts to evade responsibility for regulating the use of small boats." I don't know if it was a result of the jury's recommendation and all the publicity from this case, but the federal government quietly shelved their plan to change the regulations regarding life jackets in small boats.

Safety in the construction industry was another area where I thought the Coroner's Office could bring pressure for improvement. During the postwar years Toronto became a boom city and construction in and around the area increased twenty-fold. In their rush to get the new buildings erected, contractors began cutting corners wherever possible and one of those places was in the area of safety. The craft unions were tightly organized and took steps to protect their members; but most labourers did not belong to any union and the labourers' unions that were in existence were very weak and could do little for their members.

Thus some builders found that it was cheaper not to shore their excavations properly. After all, most trenches did not collapse and those that did only occasionally produced a fatality. It was true a few deaths did result, but that was considered one of the accepted hazards of the construction industry. Actually every summer from 1952 through 1962 from six to ten newly immigrated Italian labourers died in just this way, buried under an avalanche of dirt, and no one cared. Well, almost no one. At that time the Toronto *Telegram* had a hard-hitting labour reporter named Frank Drea, and he began a series of articles demanding a stop to these unnecessary deaths.

Every coroner agreed with Drea, for there was no more horrible experience than having to go to the flat of some immigrant family to tell them that the father had been killed. I know that at least one coroner, perhaps to salve his conscience, used to give each bereaved wife a wallet full of money which he said had been found in the dead man's pocket.

It seemed to me that this was an excellent place for the Coroner's Office to carry out its function, and I instructed my staff that in future all construction deaths were to have an inquest, preceded by a thorough investigation.

We did not have long to wait. The summer of 1963 produced its usual quota of collapsing excavations, but this time every death was probed to find out who was responsible. Contractors both large and small were involved and the coroners' juries began to bring in tough recommendations. They recommended that contractors be forced to hire full-time inspectors, that they be forced to post safety bonds, that the prime contractor be required to accept full responsibility for safety in his projects, and most important, that criminal charges be laid when failure to follow safety regulations had been proved.

By the end of that summer all the Toronto newspapers had made these trench collapses and inquests front-page news and they now began to run editorials demanding governmental action. The *Star* led the attack: "This metropolis has had too much of carelessness and bloodshed in building and tunnelling. There have been two royal commissions in the last 3 years — and still there are sloppy methods, feckless employers taking shortcuts, slipshod overseers. The coroner's jury recommended that criminal action be taken against the subcontracting firm. That is proper."

That did it. A provincial election was imminent and the government did not like this type of publicity. The Minister of Labour ordered his inspectors to crack down on all construction sites and to ensure that every regulation was followed, particularly in respect to shoring. And so as quickly and simply as that excavations stopped collapsing and immigrant labourers stopped dying in them. The contractors had now found it had become cheaper to shore excavations than to suffer the penalties of government fines, bad publicity, stop-work orders and criminal charges. That situation prevails to this day.

After working for some four months I found that I liked my job and expected I would spend the rest of my life at it; so I applied to join the Metropolitan Toronto employees pension plan. The personnel department of the municipality wrote me back on July 16 turning me down because they said that I was not in their employ and that they only paid me as a convenience but in actual fact I worked for the provincial government. I then wrote the provincial pension committee asking if I could contribute to their plan and they wrote back that I most certainly was not a provincial employee and it was their understanding that I worked for Metro.

Although I was then nonplussed, as the months passed and I got into increasing hot water with both levels of government I became more and more pleased by my ambiguous situation. I calculated, quite incorrectly, that if neither of them were my employer neither of them could fire me.

5 The Cancer Quacks

In the mid-1930s a Dr. Hett opened a clinic in Toronto for the purpose of treating cancer. Hett was a flamboyant quack who promised a cure to those afflicted with inoperable carcinomas if they would just receive his expensive weekly injections. I remember seeing Hett in late 1936 when he arrived at my grandmother's home in west Toronto. She was then dying of stomach cancer and my parents had called in Hett in a last desperate attempt to save her. I was then only eleven and I never forgot the impressive manner of that renegade doctor. Everyone we knew then was poor but he arrived in a chauffeur-driven limousine,wearing a black cloak which he swept off with a flourish to reveal a tuxedo and white tie. He only came to see Grandmother once and he offered to cure her for $2000, but four days later, while the family was still trying to raise the money, she died.

The very next year the College of Physicians and Surgeons investigated Hett's activities. They discovered that his magic injections were a mixture of liver and opium which undoubtedly made their recipients feel better temporarily but of course could not affect the course of their disease. The college held a hearing and ordered Hett's medical licence revoked. They never carried out their order because the then Ontario Premier Mitchell Hepburn was an admirer and friend of Hett's and he threatened the college that if they did not change their decision the government would revoke their licensing powers. Hepburn was at that time all-powerful in Ontario and the college did not dare defy him so Hett kept his licence and continued to prey on the sick and the gullible until his death several years later.

Because of their fright at Hepburn's threats, for the next twenty-six years the College of Physicians apparently made no further attemps to control any of Ontario's cancer quacks and when I was appointed Chief Coroner in 1963 I found that these men were still flourishing in Toronto. I determined to drive them out but soon found that my activities in that field brought me into direct conflict with the authorities at Queen's Park. It was not that anyone there approved of cancer quacks, but the Supervising Coroner and the Deputy Attorney General and his assistants seemed more concerned with legal niceties, and from the beginning distrusted me and my methods. Dr. Cotnam illustrated his feelings when he wrote to the Attorney General about me shortly after my appointment as Chief Coroner, "As I am sure you are aware, this type of person can be very dangerous at times. They try to put you on the spot regardless of what decision is aimed at."

In 1963 the leading medical cancer quack in Toronto was one Dr. Thomas Glover, an elderly physician who for forty-four years had been injecting his special brand of horse serum into persons he believed to be suffering from cancer. The serum itself was harmless but the false hopes it gave cancer sufferers encouraged them not to take standard medical or surgical treatment and thus in many cases led to their premature deaths. Way back in 1921 Toronto's Academy of Medicine had investigated Dr. Glover's serum and found it useless, but the doctor had rejected their findings and continued his activities unhindered. He was now eighty years of age but still carried on his active medical practice in the "treatment" of cancer.

On August 11, 1963, Mrs. Elizabeth George died shortly after admission to the Humber Memorial Hospital. Her death was investigated by Dr. Donald Bunt, one of my coroners, who recommended that an inquest be held. The circumstances were typical of other cases that had preceded hers over the years. Mrs. George had developed a cancer in her breast several years earlier and her family doctor made an early diagnosis and recommended surgery. But she had heard of Dr. Glover and sought his opinion.

He advised that instead of surgery she should receive regular injections of his serum. She followed his advice for four years until 1967, when her condition had so deteriorated that she now agreed to receive proper medical treatment. It was far too late, however, and the cancer spread through her body until she died. It was the opinion of the specialists at the hospital that had she received normal surgical treatment at the time of diagnosis she could have been cured.

This was exactly the type of case I was looking for in order to get at Dr. Glover and I seized the opportunity. For many years my predecessor had "taken over" from other coroners inquests that had interested him or which involved sensitive political topics and so I now called Dr. Bunt and told him that I would handle the inquest.

The inquest convened as ordered and the evidence that unfolded was damning. I called Dr. Glover to the stand and asked him to explain where he got his horse serum and the theory behind its use. The doctor gave a long rambling and confused story of discovering a "pleomorphic micro-organism in cancer victims which no bacteriologist can classify." He said he grew this bacteria in a fluid containing "sunflower seeds, Irish moss and Icelandic moss." He said that he then filtered the fluid and injected the bacteria into horses, "I have only 3 horses now up at Shanty Bay. I'm no authority on horses but they are healthy horses." He tested the horses' blood regularly and when he judged that "the time was right" he bled the horses and used the blood for the serum which he injected into patients. I asked him if he ever conducted autopsies to determine the effects of his serum and he replied, "No, because I didn't have much time."

Dr. Joe Dawson testified for the College of Physicians and Surgeons. He said that as a result of numerous complaints the registrar of the College of Physicians and Surgeons had recommended that Dr. Glover's practices be investigated some fifteen years earlier but that when Dr. Glover refused to appear before them the matter had been dropped.

Mrs. Irene Lock, Mrs. George's daughter, testified that her mother had had great faith in Dr. Glover and said that her mother had told her that the doctor had promised she would be kept alive as long as she was under his care.

This evidence was followed by that of a specialist in internal medicine from the University of Toronto, who gave it as his opinion that Dr. Glover's cancer treatment was useless, or worse, if it prevented cancer sufferers from receiving other treatment. At this point unfortunately we ran out of time and I adjourned the inquest to reconvene the following week. It was my hope that the jury would recommend that Dr. Glover's licence to practice should be cancelled.

Meanwhile Dr. Glover had hired a clever young lawyer who, after studying the Coroner's Act, appealed to the Supreme Court to quash the inquest under Section 10 of the Act which then read: "After the issue of the warrant no other coroner shall issue a warrant or interfere in the case except the Supervising Coroner or except under the instructions of the Attorney General or the Crown Attorney." No such instructions were of course forthcoming and the Supreme Court ordered the inquest quashed.

I was still determined that Dr. Glover must be put out of business and so instructed Dr. Bunt to order a new inquest which he should conduct himself. However, Dr. Cotnam, the Supervising Coroner, now came to the morgue and advised Dr. Bunt that "because of the evidence given on the prior inquest, no further inquest was necessary." Poor Dr. Bunt did not know what to do in this situation and so went to the Deputy Attorney General, William Common, to seek direction. Mr. Common told Dr. Bunt that he did not think that an inquest should be held for the sole purpose of exposing the unorthodox practices of Dr. Glover and I could hardly blame Dr. Bunt when he decided to drop the matter.

My feelings towards Dr. Cotnam and Mr. Common were not as charitable, but there was nothing I could then do about it. I did, however, write the College of Physicians and Surgeons and laid a charge of medical misconduct against Dr. Glover. They did not bother to answer my letter and so six months later I pressed them to take some action. Finally, another eight months later, they acted to protect the public; Dr. Glover was allowed to continue his medical practice with full privileges provided that he did not employ serum in the treatment of any cancer patient.

While this battle was proceeding, other troubles came right along with it. Just a few days after the quashing of the Elizabeth George inquest and before the college and I fell out over my pressing them to take action against Dr. Glover, Dr. Dawson of the College of Physicians and Surgeons phoned me to say that he was very pleased with the manner in which I had handled Dr. Glover and that since the college was unable to get at these men would I be willing to look at another case. He told me the story of Margaret Power.

This young lady had received a routine medical examination at the Toronto Western Hospital in March of 1960; a cancer was suspected and she was advised to have surgery. She refused and went to see a Dr. Leo Roy, who promised a cure without surgery and for the next year treated her with health foods, a short-wave electrical machine and serum injections. On her deathbed in the spring of 1962 Miss Power wrote a lengthy statement detailing the treatment she had received from Dr. Roy, the promises he had made and the moneys she had paid him. She wrote that the last line of a speech the doctor had made would always be in her memory. He had allegedly declared: "Surgery is no cure for cancer." She also wrote that Dr. Roy had "quoted statistics that surgery cured 5 percent of cancer, nature cured 7 percent and his treatments cured 80 percent." Miss Power died at home in May 1962 and was buried with no autopsy being performed or coroner being called. It was not until the following March that Miss Power's mother took her daughter's statement to the authorities and this resulted in the college approaching me to request that an inquest be held.

I was in a bit of a quandary because no inquest may be ordered by a coroner without first viewing the body of the deceased and this had not been done. The Attorney General may, however, order an inquest without such a viewing having taken place. So I went to the office of Fred Cass to seek his permission. I did not see Mr. Cass but was interviewed by his deputy, Bill Common, who by now made little effort to hide his disapproval of my activities. He flatly refused me permission for the inquest, giving three reasons: first, it was a problem for the college and was none of my business; second, more than a year had passed since the death of Miss Power; and third, I had already upset the medical profession with the George inquest.

I was now becoming used to stepping around the obstacles in

the Attorney General's department. I called a press conference at which I released the results of my investigation, warned the public not to visit Dr. Roy and said that I intended to lay charges of medical misconduct against him with the college. (Coroners had no special privileges or responsibilities in the matter of medical misconduct of other physicians, but I felt that since a death had resulted I should take some action.) The doctor roared "libel" and threatened to sue but nothing came of this and on August 21, 1964 the college acted on my complaint and took away Dr. Roy's licence to practise.

Simultaneously with my battles with Drs. Glover and Roy I took on a non-medical man who had a "cure" for cancer. On September 30, 1963, I received a telephone call from a Mr. Philip Podoliak whose wife was dying of cancer. I visited Mrs. Podoliak and took a statement from her. She said that the previous April she had learned of a Dr. V. Mirkovich, a Ph.D. in chemistry, who claimed to have a serum cure for cancer. Mirkovich had negotiated with the Podoliaks and had demanded $100,000 for his treatment and presence. They had been unable to raise this huge amount and no treatment had been given; but for several weeks Mrs. Podoliak had discontinued her regular medical treatments while she pleaded with Mirkovich.

After Mrs. Podoliak's death on December 27, 1963, I wrote to Attorney General Cass pointing out that no other governmental body had the power to take any action against Mirkovich and requested permission to hold an inquest. Mr. Cass ordered a report from his officials who advised him that "there appears to be nothing illegal in the conduct of Dr. Mirkovich." I was refused permission to hold an inquest and once again gave the facts to the press. No charges were ever laid but Mirkovich did cease his activities and disappeared from public view in this country.

Now that I look back ten years later, it is perfectly clear that these conflicts with the Attorney General's department came from two entirely different concepts of the purpose of a coroner and an inquest. I had read all the relevant books and concluded that there was only one real purpose for an inquest and that was to prevent similar deaths in the future. The officials of the government, however, had read the Coroner's Act and they knew that the purpose of an inquest was solely to determine the cause of death—the where, when and how.

I am happy to say that although it took nine years and uncounted fights, I finally won this war. In 1972, five years after I had been fired as Chief Coroner, the government introduced a new Coroner's Act setting out that the purpose of an inquest is to prevent similar deaths in the future. I am also very proud that since 1964 I have known of no cancer quacks practising in Ontario.

6 *Slapped Down by the Supreme Court*

The Shouldice Clinic in Toronto is a world-famous private hospital specializing in the treatment of hernias. The clinic's founder, Dr. Earl Shouldice, had developed a highly successful operation for this condition which was done under local anaesthetic and resulted in a lower recurrence rate than is found anywhere else in the world.

On July 10, 1963, seventy-one-year old Horace Burnett died at the clinic following an operation for a hernia the previous day. The investigating coroner, Dr. Elie Cass, told me of his findings and recommended that an inquest be held because in his opinion physical conditions at the hospital appeared deficient. I told him to go ahead and it was booked for September 11, 1963.

A few days before the inquest was to be held I was visited at my home by the former mayor of Toronto, Nathan Phillips who, as a lawyer, had been engaged by Dr. Shouldice to represent him at the inquest. Phillips expressed some apprehension about Cass's attitude, saying that Dr. Shouldice felt that he was hostile to him. Phillips asked if I would mind sitting in at the inquest with Dr. Cass to ensure that Dr. Shouldice was fairly treated and so as to reassure him. This was not an unusual request, as my predecessor, Smirle Lawson had often sat on the bench with new coroners to guide them and I did not hesitate in following the same procedure.

The inquest itself was very thorough and I felt that Dr. Cass conducted it entirely fairly. I sat beside him and did not interfere in any way but confined myself to a few clarifying questions. Dr. Shouldice did not like the jury's verdict at all; they did not question his clinic's competence but they were very unhappy with its facilities. They recommended that patients be given a more intensive examination before an operation, that the hospital have a certified anaesthetist available and present during operations, that the hospital have a resident doctor to handle emergencies and that the hospital be equipped with a complete range of breathing tubes and other equipment.

Dr. Shouldice now changed lawyers and his new lawyer appealed to the Supreme Court of Ontario to quash the inquest and its findings on the grounds that I had acceded to the request of Dr. Shouldice's first lawyer and sat in on the inquest! To my amazement not only did Mr. Justice Edward Richardson quash the inquest on those grounds but he also went on to say "The inquest was unnecessary especially since Dr. Shouldice enjoys such a tremendous reputation. I don't agree that any mistake was made at the hospital but if one was it should have been taken up by the College of Physicians and Surgeons. There would be ten inquests a day if one was called every time a patient died in a hospital." The judge was especially unhappy about the jury's recommendations: "It's not a matter for a lay jury to decide. It is outside their scope to make recommendations of this nature." He finished by saying that I "would be better advised to read the Coroner's Act than to be ordering inquests into deaths at hospitals" and as his final shot he refused me the usual order protecting a government official from civil proceedings.

I could not understand how any judge could come to these conclusions—after all, not only had he not heard the evidence at the inquest, he had not even had the opportunity to see a transcript. I decided that his decision had to be appealed, for the whole purpose of an inquest was now called into question.

I wrote to Attorney General Cass requesting permission to appeal the judgment of Mr. Justice Richardson but the Attorney General replied saying that he agreed with the judge and he refused me permission to appeal. Two months later Dr. Shouldice appeared on television to announce that he had no intention of following the jury's recommendations.

On December 16, 1964, I wrote the following letter to Dr. Shouldice:

> Dear Dr. Shouldice:
>
> It is now exactly one year since the inquest into the death of Horace Burnett was quashed. Once an inquest is quashed it legally did not occur and it would have been quite proper for me to order Dr. Cass to hold a new inquest in the case.
>
> Until now I have not done so in order to avoid further unfavourable publicity for your clinic and in the hope that you would carry out several of the jury's recommendations to improve your equipment and pre-operative technique.
>
> I feel sufficient time has now passed to make a final decision and I would therefore request your reply as to which of the jury's recommendations you have carried out or intend to carry out.
>
> Please be assured that I do not wish to cause you unnecessary difficulties but it was the opinion of the independent expert called as a witness that changes were essential at your surgery. I am anxious to prevent future unnecessary mortality.
> Please advise me at your earliest convenience.

I did not receive a reply from Dr. Shouldice but I did receive a telephone call from Frank Wilson, the Assistant Deputy Attorney General, who advised me that Dr. Shouldice had been in contact with Premier Robarts and that Mr. Arthur Wishart, the new Attorney General, had instructed Wilson to phone me and tell me to stop bothering Dr. Shouldice. (I didn't learn it till much later but Dr. Shouldice had written a letter to the Premier in which he called me a "self appointed McCarthyite" and "a psychopathic personality who instantly publicizes himself as the great emancipator of the medical profession and hospitals in Ontario and should be removed from his position of persecution.")

My secretary recorded the conversation with Frank Wilson, which went as follows:

Wilson: Listen, I didn't spoil your Hanukkah, how come you're spoiling my Christmas?

Shulman: What do you mean?
Wilson: That letter you sent to Dr. Shouldice, he has been in touch with the Premier and Mr. Wishart told me to tell you to cause no further trouble to Dr. Shouldice.
Shulman: I don't want to cause Dr. Shouldice any trouble but will you ask him to bring in some of the recommendations made by the jury to bring his hospital up to scratch and that will be the end of the matter.
Wilson: We will see.

A month later I wrote to Dr. Shouldice again.

> Dear Dr. Shouldice:
>
> It is now five weeks since I wrote to you and although I have not received a reply from you I did get a phone call from an official at the Attorney General's Department expressing displeasure that I had followed up the case.
>
> I am very disappointed that rather than make those simple changes at the clinic which could prevent future deaths, you would attempt to silence me through the Attorney General's Department.
>
> Despite this incident, I am still willing to forego holding an inquest to replace the quashed one provided that I receive an assurance from you that at least a portion of the jury's recommendations have been carried out or will be carried out.
>
> I trust that I will receive a more direct reply to this letter.

Once again there was no direct reply from Dr. Shouldice but I did receive a letter from the Attorney General in which he said: "In my opinion this letter to Dr. Shouldice constitutes a threat that if Dr. Shouldice does not comply with a jury's verdict which has no legal effect whatsoever, then Dr. Shouldice may be subjected to a further inquest with attendant unfavourable publicity. This type of threat by a public servant to a responsible member of our society is, in my opinion inexcusable, and is inconsistent with your duties as Chief Coroner."

That was the end of that particular battle but the decade since then has changed the attitude of everyone concerned. Now it is taken for granted that coroners' juries will investigate unusual hospital deaths, and their recommendations are never disregarded. It is remarkable how yesterday's controversy has become today's orthodoxy.

7 My First Firing — 1963

If all these fights were aggravating me, they were apparently upsetting the Tory politicians even more and after only six months in office the government decided they had to get rid of me. Deputy Attorney General Bill Common fired the first shot on October 1, 1963, by announcing that the post of Chief Coroner was to be abolished and my duties would be taken over by Supervising Coroner Beatty Cotnam. Mr. Common said that the change would be made in an amendment to the Ontario Coroner's Act which would be introduced in the legislature by Attorney General Fred Cass. Mr. Cass was discreetly unavailable for comment.

Dr. Cotnam made haste to voice his approval.

> I concur in this decision. I have never seen eye to eye with Dr. Shulman. This fellow has a remarkable ability to distort the truth. He has constantly refused to accept advice or instructions. If all 420 coroners thought that way there would be chaos. He's been smearing the reputation of 6500 doctors in Ontario and this of course includes all his own coroners. I don't think an inquest should be used as an instrument of persecution. He pictures himself as a Sir Galahad on a white horse trying to clean up all corruption at once. I can't accept that.

I responded with the only weapon I had. I called a press conference and asked for a full public inquiry into "political and professional interference with the operation of the Ontario coroners' system." The debate quickly degenerated into name-calling, with Bill Common denying my allegations, "I don't like to use the word 'liar'," he said. Dr. Cotnam put it more gently, "There is no place for Dr. Shulman in the long range plan of the department."

The response from the Toronto papers and the public was reassuring. Remarkably, all three papers ran editorials the next day demanding that I not be fired. (The *Star* headed their editorial "Don't Shoot the Coroner") and this was followed by literally hundreds of letters to the papers and to Premier John Robarts asking that my job be saved. These came from a general public cross-section ranging from non-political personalities like Gregory Clark and Anglican Minister Rev. S. G. West to political figures including well-known Conservatives like Stan Frolick and the former Attorney General Kelso Roberts.

In face of all this unwonted controversy Attorney General Cass beat a strategic retreat. He told the legislature on January 27, 1964, that "Dr. Shulman will be offered every opportunity to present his allegations respecting the operations of the coroners' jury system". He went on that he would not fire me "because that's a job for the civil service." He definitely ruled out a public inquiry but said that a meeting would be called in his office when all concerned could present their side of the controversy.

The three Toronto papers continued to press my case, with the *Star* once again taking the lead as they wrote, "We believe Dr. Shulman is the kind of coroner the public needs, even if he is not the kind the Attorney General's Department wants."

Premier John Robarts had had enough of this bad publicity and now advised the Attorney General to cool the matter out and to that end I was summoned to a meeting with my antagonists in Fred Cass's office on February 3, 1964. The meeting itself proved to be anti-climactic low comedy. Because of my fears of being misquoted after such a meeting I asked the Attorney General if I could bring someone with me and he agreed to this, but the question was who. I didn't want to take a lawyer because I felt this tended to make me look defensive or guilty and so finally I took along my secretary Ann Worobec.

When we arrived Mr. Cass was sitting at his long desk and

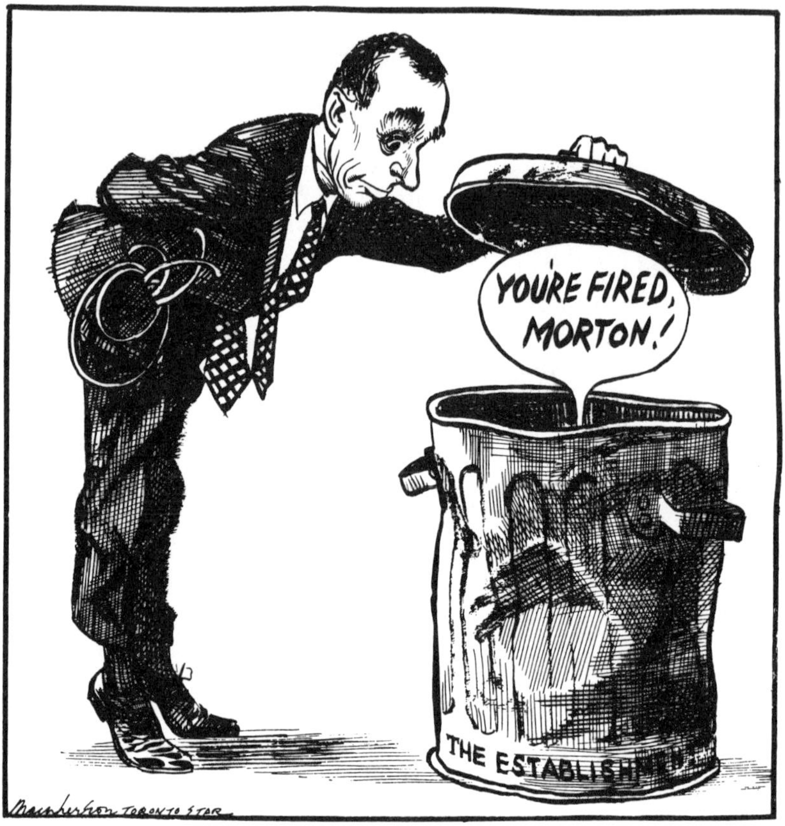

around the room in a circle he had placed his entire staff, including Dr. Cotnam and Mr. Common. Ann and I were seated in the centre of this ring and I was invited to present my side of the story, but first the Attorney General asked if we minded being searched for a tape recorder. I found the request a little strange but agreed and asked Ann to empty her purse and offered to be searched myself. At this point Mr. Cass laughed and said: "Never mind, I'll take your word for it." For the next hour I presented the material which documented all the troubles I had had with his staff in the Pisecny case and the various hospital deaths.

While I detailed all this no one spoke and when I had completed my speech Mr. Cass said, "I am going to ask Dr. Cotnam and Mr. Common to consider all these matters and prepare their replies which they will give at a second meeting. Meanwhile I will ask my deputy from the civil side, Randall Dick, to comment because he has had no connection with any of these matters." We all turned to the slight, bespectacled deputy who rose, coughed and then asked, "Dr. Shulman, didn't you once go to North Toronto Collegiate?" I nodded yes and he came over to me, pumped my hand, and said, "So did I."

So ended the great meeting; the second meeting which was to follow never took place, for the Attorney General wanted to hear no more of this whole mess and my job was now temporarily safe. Anyway that controversy was completely forgotten in the much more noisy one that followed — the Patricia Morgan case.

8 *The Patricia Morgan Case*

I thought that it was just another nut letter. Ever since I had begun to receive publicity as Toronto's Chief Coroner there had poured in requests for investigations of deaths that had taken place thirty years before, demands for help against sinister influences who were directing electrical rays at the writer, people who believed they had a cure for cancer — they seemed endless.

This particular letter which I received on January 30, 1964, was from a Ruth Neate, who wrote that her sister, Miss Patricia Morgan, had died at the East General Hospital eighteen days after an operation and Mrs. Neate felt the situation warranted an inquest. She explained why:

> I have been told that the autopsy revealed forceps in the intestine which caused shock which was the immediate cause of death. This, together with certain other information which has been given to me, forces me to make this request.

My internship had been taken at the East General Hospital some thirteen years earlier and I knew the chief pathologist, Dr. S. F. Penney, very well; so I picked up the phone and called him at the hospital. I read Ruth Neate's letter to him and before I asked him anything he said, "Yes, it's true." I was astonished and asked him why he hadn't reported the death to my office. He replied that he did not think that it was his responsibility, that he had reported his findings to both the attending surgeon, Dr. Ken Brown, who had performed the operation and the hospital authorities, and that it was their decision not to report the matter. He offered to supply me immediately with a copy of his report.

I now ordered a copy of Pat Morgan's death certificate and discovered that it made no mention of an instrument being found in the abdomen, but blamed the death on cancer—yet Dr. Penney had found no cancer during the autopsy. The death certificate was signed by Dr. Ken Brown.

My surprise up to that point was mild compared to what I felt after I spoke to Dr. Brown, for he told me an incredible tale. He said that part way through the operation he had been interrupted and harassed by a senior hospital surgeon as a result of which he (Brown) had abandoned the operation and left the operating room and that the operation had then been completed by a third doctor. Dr. Brown told me that if any instrument had been left in Pat Morgan's abdomen it had not been left by him and he went on to say that he felt it was the responsibility of the hospital administration to report the death to the Coroner's Office. His final remark unnerved me: "I used to be a journeyman stereotyper and I may have to go back to it!"

It still didn't make sense how an eight-inch forceps could be left behind in an operation: surely the surgeons counted their instruments before and after? But I soon discovered that the opposite was true—not only the East General but most Toronto hospitals did not bother to count. Furthermore, the law was very clear: section 16 of the Coroner's Act read, "Every person who has reason to believe that a deceased person died as a result of negligence, misconduct, malpractice . . . shall report the circumstances to the coroner." I had more than enough material to justify an investigation and possible charges and so I dumped the whole mess in Attorney General Cass's lap and simultaneously leaked the basic facts to the newspapers. (I did not have the power to order an inquest myself because I had not "viewed the body.") Even I was surprised at the results—front-page stories, editorials all over the province, questions in the legislature. Mr. Cass had no choice but to order an inquest, but he did not allow me to conduct it and instead placed Coroner Gerald Blanchet in charge.

Compared with what was coming, my trouble with doctors because of the publicity from the cancer quacks and the Shouldice

Clinic cases was nothing. I now learned that I was really in hot water with the entire medical profession who rallied around their beleaguered colleagues.

The public was treated to a series of newspaper articles explaining why it would be unhealthy for patients if doctors wasted time counting instruments, why inquests should not be held into hospital deaths, and even why coroners should not investigate them. Dr. Frederick Kergin, chief surgeon at the Toronto General Hospital and head of the department of surgery at the University of Toronto, was quoted as saying, "A count would slow things down to the danger of the patient. A count just isn't practical and I know of no major hospital where it is carried out." Dr. James Bateman, surgeon-in-chief at the Orthopedic and Arthritic Hospital didn't want coroners going into hospitals at all. "It would be witch-hunting in surgery and reprehensible if someone's going to stand over surgeons all the time. Hospitals should conduct their own investigations. Medical disciplinary machinery is there ready to function at all times." Dr. W. Ross Walters, chief of staff at the Salvation Army's Grace Hospital, felt that inquiries should be left to the College of Physicians and Surgeons. Sidney Liswood, administrator of the New Mount Sinai Hospital was distressed "that public confidence in hospitals may be shaken." One surgeon pointed out that coroners are usually only general practitioners. "There is a feeling of nausea about individuals presuming to dictate to people who are better qualified."

The doctors may have been aghast at my actions but the public was appalled at theirs and there was an avalanche of letters to my office, each bearing another medical gothic horror story — the result of the many years during which the profession had refused to hear the public's complaints. The following letter is a typical but particularly moving example of the mail I received:

February 26/1964

Dear Dr. Shulman:

On Dec. 13/1939, my sister, Edna Young, died in the Toronto General Hospital of double pneumonia. She had been operated on about four weeks before her death, for exophthalmic goitre. During the operation, the surgeon had severed her carotid artery. The weeks that followed were taken up with measures to save her life . . . large casts, tracheotomy, etc. but of course, it proved hopeless.

I was then twenty-one, newly married and in a state of confusion in trying to cope with my parents who were in a state of shock, disbelief and grief. My father's grief took the form of rage and injustice; my mother, Polish-born, was in despair and threatened to commit suicide. . . . The head of the College of Physicians and Surgeons called me in to see him, to try to persuade me to bring some reason to my parents. He likened her death to that of breaking a set of expensive china, which I found to be not a very consoling thought. At that time, I had been a Catholic. I lost my faith and gave up my religion, nor have I regained my faith at any time since then.

My father read what he could about goitre operations and then insisted on seeing the case history. After finding out what had happened, he went to see a criminal lawyer in this city, and although he said he did have a case of negligence, that it would be impossible to bring a charge against the medical profession. We were very poor at that time, and it would have taken a great deal of money, so he took the lawyer's advice and gave up the idea.

You may well imagine, then, the intense interest I have in the present inquest. It is not so much that those surviving members want revenge against the doctors who are to blame; but the old cry: "We want the truth and we want justice." To compound the error by concealing the facts, is heartless. Whatever the outcome of the inquest, there will only be bitterness in the hearts of those who must live with the knowledge of the error until they die, as I must do and as my mother must do.

This letter is written to express to you as well, my admiration for your position in this matter and for the strength of principle you have shown. How I wish you had been in this position in 1939 . . . or someone like you.

Whether you answer this letter or not is up to you; but I wanted to write it to let you know that such a tragedy is never erased, is never corrected or made right again; but one does need the highest consideration and above all the truth.

Your sincerely,
Irma Coucill

The Patricia Morgan inquest itself went on for days and two extraordinary but radically different stories came out. Dr. Brown on the one hand described the operation as one which could well have been successful but which was interfered with and ultimately mishandled by doctors both junior and senior to him.

Dr. Ken Brown was forty-five, an apparently successful surgeon who had struggled to put himself through medical school, had served in the army and taken four years of post-graduate medical training. His life had been marred by a tragic incident in which he had been treated with a new antibiotic to cure a minor finger infection but the antibiotic had previously unknown side effects and had damaged Dr. Brown's hearing. For eight years he had done all his surgical work at the East General Hospital, but he was not part of the regular hospital staff and was looked on with some suspicion by the rest of the operating team.

The chief surgeon at the hospital, Dr. Burns Plewes, was sixty years old, tall, distinguished and grey. He had been called to the East General fourteen years before to take over and upgrade the department of surgery from the general practitioners of limited competence who had built, organized and run the hospital. His ability was unquestioned but it was an open secret at the hospital that he found it personally distasteful and often impossible to clamp down on the many incompetent physicians still on staff at the East General. For two years Dr. Plewes had had grave doubts about Ken Brown's surgical abilities but instead of denying him operating privileges he had made a practice of assigning surgical assistants as a safeguard at all Dr. Brown's operations. One of these was an eager twenty-six-year-old, Dr. A.T. Varga, the hospital's senior surgical resident who had been ordered to assist and watch Dr. Brown in his operation on Pat Morgan.

Self-assured, young, stocky and darkly handsome, Dr. Varga was an absolute contrast to Dr. Brown in both appearance and manner. He believed the operation had been mishandled by Dr. Brown from the start and, at the inquest, made little effort to hide his feelings of contempt towards Dr. Brown's surgical ability. Varga had graduated from the University of Toronto medical school in 1958 and had subsequently trained further at several Toronto hospitals including the Banting Institute and the Toronto

General. In July 1963 he had become chief resident at the East General Hospital. His duties included overseeing all the interns and arranging all assistants for surgery in the operating room, looking after all public ward patients for surgery, being on call for surgical emergencies at all times and deciding who should leave the intensive care unit when it was full and a bed was needed for someone else.

Relations between Dr. Brown and Dr. Varga were strained before they undertook the Patricia Morgan operation. They had had an argument during a previous operation when Dr. Varga had expressed doubts about the surgical method which Dr. Brown had been following. Certainly there was no question that Dr. Varga felt that Dr. Brown was not a competent surgeon, while Dr. Brown felt he knew far more about surgery than Varga possibly could and looked upon him as an unavoidable annoyance.

Patricia Morgan had first come to Dr. Brown in December 1961 complaining of stomach pains. Medical treatment had not helped and her condition worsened and so Dr. Brown had operated on her in March 1963 and discovered cancer of the stomach. He removed much of her stomach and hoped he had cured her. Unfortunately after a few months Miss Morgan's symptoms recurred and X-rays revealed that she had a completely obstructed bowel.

All the doctors involved felt that Pat Morgan had had a recurrence of her cancer, that it had spread and that she was probably dying. Dr. Brown was anxious to operate on her a second time in an attempt to relieve the obstruction even though he was advised against doing so by other East General Hospital doctors, especially Dr. Burns Plewes, who had urged him to accept the situation that his patient was incurably ill of cancer. After the ill-fated operation Dr. Brown insisted that he had never been convinced that the cancer had recurred and he believed that the operation would reveal what was really wrong.

When he prepared for the operation Dr. Brown found that Dr. Varga and Dr. Paul Takahashi, a surgical intern, had been assigned to "assist" him. The mutual antipathy between Dr. Brown and Dr. Varga was evident throughout the operation and led to a series of quarrels during the ordeal.

Doctors Varga and Takahashi met Dr. Brown in the hall before the operation. While they scrubbed Dr. Brown told them the case history. When they entered the operating room Dr. Brown took a position on the right side of the patient, Dr. Takahashi on Brown's left, and Dr. Varga on the opposite side of the table. At the patient's head was Dr. Coggins, the anaesthetist, whose responsibilities included maintaining the patient's breathing and blood pressure during the operation.

According to Dr. Brown's testimony at the inquest, there was trouble almost at once. Soon after opening the abdomen Dr. Brown was amazed when Dr. Varga began to show him a process of cleaning tissue from membranes which Dr. Brown had learned in medical school and had known well for many years. The usual procedure is for the operating surgeon to do any teaching to his assistants, not vice versa. Dr. Brown stated, "I was surprised but I let it go. It was a bit of a nuisance and an annoyance but I didn't make an issue of it. I ignored it."

The operation proceeded very slowly. As a result of the previous operation, considerable scar tissue had formed in the abdomen and this had to be carefully dissected away in order to expose the blockage in the intestine. There was no sign of cancer.

As Dr. Brown began working in the area of the spleen, he noticed that Dr. Varga was becoming quite concerned. The spleen, an organ which creates, stores and destroys blood, is a sensitive one which doctors normally try to avoid disturbing, although a person can live quite well without it. Despite Dr. Varga's objections, Dr. Brown proceeded and accidentally cut through a small artery creating a moderate amount of steady bleeding. Dr. Brown felt that the blood loss was minimal and was not alarmed but, according to his testimony, "At the onset of bleeding Dr. Varga left the operation, my assistant disappeared!" Then, after a few minutes Dr. Varga returned and, Dr. Brown said, again began dissecting, now working on the opposite side of the operating table from Dr. Brown. From this position Dr. Brown felt that Varga could not see where he was working. Dr. Brown said that he objected to his assistant's dissection and that Dr. Varga replied, "Dr. Brown! I insist!" Dr. Brown, the surgeon in charge of the operation, said that Varga was dissecting for about one and a half hours, much of it without his permission. "I withdrew permission when it became obvious that his roughness was to the detriment of the patient."

Then, Dr. Brown said, Dr. Varga had injured the capsule surrounding the spleen by "rough dissection." Once a spleen is injured, bleeding can rarely if ever be controlled and invariably it must be removed. As could be expected, blood rapidly began to ooze from the damaged spleen. This flow of blood in addition to the previous cuts made further progress difficult, and began to endanger the life of the patient.

At this point Dr. Varga went to the door of the operating room and asked the nurse to call Dr. Burns Plewes. Within minutes Dr. Plewes arrived and began to speak to Dr. Brown, mentioning both his concern about the bleeding and his feeling that Miss Morgan, with her history of abdominal cancer, would not likely survive long after the operation.

In later discussions with Dr. Plewes, Dr. Brown stressed that he felt he could have cleared up the obstruction that he believed was causing Miss Morgan's trouble if Dr. Plewes had let him finish. This he felt would have been better than letting the patient starve because she could not keep her food down.

Dr. Plewes had replied that the patient would have to be fed by tube for the rest of her life. He contended this was better than proceeding with an operation once the patient had suffered a severe blood loss of the kind that Miss Morgan had experienced. From his long surgical experience he felt certain that if the operation had been continued she would have died on the table.

Dr. Brown testified that he had stopped the bleeding by this time but was forced to divert his attention from the patient to his discussion with Dr. Plewes. Dr. Brown told Dr. Plewes that he believed that the patient was young enough to stand a good chance of recovery and that there had been no evidence of cancer recurrence.

"Despite all I could say, Dr. Plewes was still convinced of his judgment," Dr. Brown said. "Only after twenty minutes did the doctor giving the patient the anaesthetic find it necessary to give her a second blood transfusion through the leg in addition to the one she was getting in the arm. At this time Dr. Plewes noticed there was considerable bleeding in the cavity. I said the patient had been bleeding during all the talking. I tried to stop it. I was still alone. Dr. Plewes asked if I wouldn't like a little assistance. I said I would very much. Then Dr. Varga returned to the operating table. Dr. Plewes said I must remove the spleen to stop the bleeding. Dr. Varga started to remove it but was having difficulty, so Dr. Plewes said he would scrub up and help."

Dr. Brown said that Dr. Plewes now left to scrub up. Dr. Brown offered to show Dr. Varga how to remove the spleen. Several large clamps were now applied to stop the blood flowing to the spleen. These were in addition to other clamps applied elsewhere earlier by Doctors Brown, Varga and Takahashi.

"The spleen was removed in less than two minutes, before Dr. Plewes returned," Dr. Brown said, "and all the bleeding was stopped. There wasn't enough room in the cavity for all the people there. I turned around to rinse my gloves before completing the closure. Dr. Varga stepped into my place at the operating table and said he would complete the operation."

Dr. Brown felt that all there was left to do was to replace the displaced organs and close the incision. He allowed Dr. Varga to complete the procedure rather than force another argument. "So I left."

The operation had thus been completed without achieving its purpose which was to expose and relieve the obstruction. Far worse was the fact that the cancer had already been completely removed in the first operation and Pat Morgan might have lived—except that an eight-inch forceps had been left behind in her abdomen.

Dr. Tony Varga's testimony at the inquest differed strikingly from Dr. Brown's account of the operation from beginning to end. He testified that he had received his first instructions about the Morgan operation from his chief, Dr. Plewes, on October 17th. Burns Plewes instructed him "to take able assistants" with him. Normally Dr. Varga would have assigned a senior and junior intern to the case but following these instructions decided to go himself and take Dr. Takahashi as his assistant.

Dr. Varga had made one thing clear to Dr. Plewes. He told him, "I would not interfere or take over this case because of previous experience (with Dr. Brown). I wanted to make certain Dr. Plewes would be in the hospital. I would assist but I would not take over although I would call Dr. Plewes if severity merited, that is, if the patient was in danger."

Dr. Varga said that by the word "interfere" he meant "doing any part of the surgical procedure himself against Dr. Brown's wishes."

Dr. Varga said the initial incision to enter the abdominal cavity took a long time because the previous operation had produced a lot of scar tissue. He denied Dr. Brown's statements that he had interfered by teaching Dr. Brown at this point. "I don't recall doing any part of this incision although I might have."

He said there were many adhesions which Dr. Brown started to separate. While doing so, Dr. Brown made a hole in the jejunum, the section of the small intestine closest to the stomach, but Dr. Varga said that such damage is not unusual while dividing adhesions.

As Dr. Brown continued with the dissection Dr. Varga said he got up into "the left side of the abdomen where I could not see. Therefore, I changed positions with Dr. Takahashi."

Dr. Varga denied doing "rough dissection" in areas where he could not see. He said that up to this stage of the operation he had not done any dissection within the cavity.

After he moved around the table Dr. Varga asked Dr. Brown to "show me the anatomy," that is to let him see into the abdominal cavity.

"I felt Dr. Plewes had sent me to make sure everything was done adequately. I felt I could not do this unless I knew the anatomy. I could not see everything from the other side of the table.

"Because of Dr. Brown's difficulty in hearing, I didn't think he heard me at first." Dr. Brown continued the dissection, so "I put out my arm to attract his attention and asked him again. He just stepped back, indicating I could look."

A disagreement then occurred when, according to Dr. Varga, he looked into the cavity and put his finger under the small bowel and said, "This is the small bowel." Dr. Varga said Dr. Brown replied that it was the colon (large bowel) which is different in appearance. "When I disagreed with him he asked, 'where is the colon?'. I showed it to him behind the small bowel." The significance of Varga's worry here was that if Dr. Brown was unable to identify the geography in the abdominal cavity, precious time was going to be wasted searching for the old operation site before the obstruction could be relieved.

Dr. Brown continued his dissection and now said he had to "mobilize" the spleen so that he could work more freely.

Dr. Varga testified that he felt the spleen was in a fairly normal position and he didn't think there was any need to take the action Dr. Brown proposed.

Dr. Varga insisted that he did not tear the capsule of the spleen as Dr. Brown said, and moreover that he had warned Dr. Brown of the danger of damaging the spleen, but Dr. Brown went ahead anyway.

Varga said that Dr. Brown "entered the capsule of the spleen with scissors." The spleen began to bleed and sponges were put over it so that the bleeding would not interfere with the vision of the surgeons.

Dr. Varga said that he cut only one adhesion in the stomach area and did not do any other dissection inside the cavity, and therefore he was not responsible for the bleeding which eventually stopped the operation.

Another disagreement soon occurred when Varga twice touched Dr. Brown on the arm and told him that what he was handling was not an adhesion but one of the membranes of the organs. Dr. Brown disagreed with him. Varga testified that he warned Brown that if he cut at this point, " 'you will have severe bleeding.' Then he cut them and there was severe bleeding."

It was after this incident that the anaesthetist, Dr. Coggins, became alarmed and said he could not obtain a blood pressure reading. He called another doctor to help administer blood and a second transfusion was set up to run simultaneously with the first one. Dr. Varga then asked Dr. Brown what he was going to do next. "He said that he was going to revise his gastrectomy. This means he was going to take more of the stomach out."

Dr. Varga believed that this would take another two hours and he felt it shouldn't be done because of the bleeding and because the patient's life was in danger. They had already spent two hours just cutting adhesions. Dr. Varga advised Dr. Brown that he should not go ahead with the gastrectomy but that he should just remove the spleen so as to control the bleeding. However Dr. Brown replied that it was essential to remove the obstruction at the stomach.

It was at this point, Dr. Varga said, that he told the nurse at the doorway to call the chief surgeon, Dr. Plewes. Varga strongly emphasized that he "did not leave."

In a few minutes Dr. Plewes arrived and Dr. Varga told him that a lot of blood had been lost, the spleen had been damaged, and the bleeding was continuing. Doctors Plewes and Brown had some conversation and Varga said he moved out of the way to let Dr. Plewes see the patient. The chief surgeon could not move in closely, however, because he was not scrubbed for the operation.

Burns Plewes gave his opinion that removal of the spleen was necessary but again Dr. Brown said that he wanted to remove the obstruction. Dr. Varga said he told his chief there was a hole in the jejunum; Dr. Brown denied this but in a few minutes he found the hole with his forceps and agreed that there was. The chief surgeon then asked Dr. Varga to feel with his fingers through the hole into the stomach. Dr. Varga did this and Dr. Plewes then said that since there was not a complete obstruction it was not absolutely vital for Miss Morgan's survival that the obstruction be removed, and that given her dangerously weakened condition, the spleen should be removed and the patient closed up. Dr. Plewes said to Dr. Brown, "Ken, you have no choice."

Dr. Varga disputed Dr. Brown's claim that Miss Morgan's blood pressure had dropped to the point where it was reported as unobtainable only during the discussion among the doctors. He said it had reached that point before he called Dr. Plewes and that is why he called him.

When Dr. Brown removed the spleen he used a method which Dr. Varga disapproved of as more difficult and dangerous. However, within a very few minutes the spleen was out and the bleeding controlled. Dr. Varga said he then asked Dr. Brown twice if he should stitch the wound and close up the patient; Dr. Brown twice replied yes but did not give up the needle holder. Dr.

Varga flatly denied Dr. Brown's statement that Dr. Varga stepped into his place at the table.

According to Dr. Varga's testimony, Dr. Brown continued to do the stitching himself until only three inches of the ten-inch incision remained open, when he finally handed over the needle and sutures to Dr. Varga. Dr. Varga started to sew up and Dr. Brown had told him the type of suture to use. Dr. Varga testified that Dr. Brown didn't remove his surgical gown, and stood looking out the window for some time.

There were, of course, a number of other people in the room—Doctors Takahashi and Coggins and several nurses. It is interesting to study their statements, as the jury had to, to try to determine what actually happened during this disastrous operation. One must bear in mind, however, that their sympathies would naturally lie with their fellow staff member, Dr. Varga, rather than the outsider, Dr. Brown. It is unfortunate that they all heard Dr. Varga's story before contributing theirs.

On one essential matter everyone agrees: before closing up the abdomen no search was made for instruments. Dr. Varga felt that this was the responsibility of Dr. Brown, the surgeon in charge, while Dr. Brown believed that when Dr. Varga took his place at the table he should and would carry out this duty.

Each man blamed the other for not seeking the forceps, but Dr. Varga claimed that he did not take over the operation until after Dr. Brown had begun to sew up the incision and this testimony was backed up by the interns and nurses also present in the operating room. Neither doctor had checked for missing instruments.

After the operation no one had the slightest idea that an instrument had been left in Pat Morgan's abdomen. She lingered for sixteen days, gradually went downhill and died on November 4, 1963. The forceps was found at the autopsy but neither the pathologist, the hospital administrator, or any of the surgeons involved reported it to my office, for they were attempting to protect the reputation of the hospital and in some cases themselves.

After hearing the conflicting testimony the coroner's jury deliberated for four and a half hours and then brought in a verdict placing the responsibility for the forceps being left behind with Dr. Brown and to the "state of disorganization" in the operating room. More important, they recommended that a count of surgical instruments be made at all operations.

An interesting side issue now came up when Dr. J. C. Dawson, registrar of the college was asked if charges of malpractice would be laid against anyone involved and he replied that the college had no power to deal with malpractice, errors of judgment or negligence by physicians.

The outcome of the Patricia Morgan case was a satisfactory one for me, for there were two major changes. Two months after the Morgan case was concluded the Canadian Medical Protective Association sent all its members a sharply worded article in which they were instructed that instrument-counting was a normal and essential procedure. Immediately all the dissenting voices became silent and counting of instruments before and after operations became standard procedure in hospitals right across Canada. The other change took a little longer, as MPP's began to urge that the government bring in legislation giving the College of Physicians power to discipline its members for malpractice or negligence. Finally, three years later the government brought in the necessary legislation.

9 *Tonsil Deaths*

The sad death of three-year-old Christopher O'Kelly led to the saving of dozens of other young lives. Up until 1964 anywhere from three to twelve children died in Toronto every year following tonsillectomies; it was considered the price to pay for the health benefits accruing to the many thousands of children who had their tonsils removed uneventfully. Each hospital had developed its own method of caring for their little patients after the operation and all but one of them had the occasional fatality.

On December 3, 1963, Christopher O'Kelly died in St. Michael's Hospital from a haemorrhage eight hours after his tonsils had been removed. The operating surgeon had not been aware that his patient was in any difficulty until just before the child died, even though the child had been taken from his bed to the examining room three times as a result of haemorrhaging. Each time the resident and senior interns had stopped the bleeding and returned the child, apparently in good condition, to his room (there was no special ward for tonsillectomy patients). After the third bleed the child went into shock and died shortly thereafter.

In the course of investigating the death Coroner Fred Cruikshank reported to me that the Hospital for Sick Children had not suffered a tonsil death for over a decade because of a strict routine which they had developed. I ordered him to pull out all stops in the inquest and to bring in experts from the Hospital for Sick

Children to testify how they avoided these disasters. Dr. Cruikshank did an excellent job in conducting the inquest and the jury followed the advice of the experts which he called, and at the conclusion of the inquest brought in the following verdict:

> We the jury recommend:
> (a) A more informative case history be made at the time of admittance, including a pre-operative haemoglobin and blood pressure reading.
> (b) A post-operative tonsil room, made available for children, under constant and continuous supervision of a nurse familiar with post-operative care.
> (c) At overt signs of bleeding the nurse in charge of the floor should be responsible for the notification of the attending physician and resident staff.
> (d) Blood sampling for cross-checking and typing to be carried out at first indication of primary bleeding.
> (e) Use of a graduated suction bottle to record the blood loss.
> (f) A child's blood pressure cuff available at all times in the tonsil room.
> (g) A set of standing orders to cover procedures for admission, assessment, operation and post-operative treatment emphasizing bleeding and shock routine.

Two days after the inquest was concluded on April 4, 1964, St. Michael's Hospital announced that they would immediately adopt all the recommendations made by the jury and within two weeks every other Toronto hospital followed suit.

Since April 4, 1964 to my knowledge no children have died in Toronto following tonsillectomy.

Later in the spring of 1964 the Coroner's Office was desperately short of room and I decided to clean out the old files in the basement and make a new office in that long unused space. Before discarding the ancient files I went through them — they were practically all old reports of coroners' investigations or inquests but there was one slim file folder marked "confidential" consisting of copies of letters my predecessor Smirle Lawson had sent out. His now deceased clerk Eddy Armour had hidden the copies in the basement for reasons we shall never know.

The folder held only six letters, two of which revealed the amiable cooperation between the Chief Coroner and the proprietor of *The Globe and Mail*. Two others demonstrated the ethnic discrimination practised with the coroner system. Eric Silk, the Deputy Attorney General had asked Dr. Lawson what work Coroner Dr. Lore was doing. Dr. Lawson had replied that many well-to-do families with a death in their home might resent being questioned by Dr. Lore, who was Chinese. Consequently all Chinese cases were assigned to Dr. Lore. Dr. Lawson said it would be impossible to say how many cases Dr. Lore would handle. (Actually he was never given a single case.)

To my amazement there was in addition an exchange of letters between Dr. Cotnam and Dr. Lawson in which Dr. Lawson had in effect advised Dr. Cotnam, then Coroner for Renfrew County, to cover up the case of an accidental death of a child there during a tonsillectomy. Dr. Cotnam had investigated the death of a three-year-old girl, Barbara Moore, who had been given a too-vigorous administration of oxygen which had ruptured her stomach. The parents of the child and the local newspaper evidently were showing increasing discontent. Dr. Cotnam asked whether there should be an inquest in this, or in all anaesthetic and surgical deaths occurring in operating rooms.

Dr. Lawson had replied as follows:

Re: Barbara Moore, Aged 3 Years (d).

> We, in Toronto, do not hold inquests in all deaths due to Anaesthetic or Surgical Deaths, as they are usually accidental.
>
> My advice to you would be to consult with your local Crown Attorney, and if he thinks an inquest should be held, then hold an inquest.
>
> In my opinion, I do not think an inquest is necessary.
>
> Thanks for writing me about this case, and also for your good work in Renfrew County, and with kindest regards to you.

I admit that this last exchange of letters gave me a feeling of indecent pleasure. After the O'Kelly inquest I had praised the jury and had remarked that if cases like this had been openly investigated in the past instead of being covered up by coroners, many lives would have been saved. Dr. Cotnam injudiciously (as it turned out) jumped on my remark to say that no cases of this type had ever been suppressed. (Of course, he had no way of knowing of the cache in the basement). Now that I had these papers in my hand I wasted no time in calling the Crown Attorney in Renfrew County to find out the disposition of the case. I discovered that not only had no inquest been held, but there had not even been an investigating report filed as is required by law and the parents had never been informed of the cause of their daughter's death.

I unkindly sent copies of these two letters both to the Supervising Coroner H. Beatty Cotnam and to his boss the new Attorney General Arthur Wishart, suggesting that amends were required. At the time it was quite irresistible, but looking back I feel some embarrassment, for Smirle Lawson ran a very tight ship and once he had given his "advice" no coroner dared disobey him. Dr. Cotnam was in no different position from any other of Smirle's subordinates.

In any case my "find" did not improve relations between the Attorney General's department and myself.

10 *Abortions*

The controversy over abortions rages on today with the Catholic Church and the "Right to Life" organization on one side saying abortions are now too easy to get, and the women's libbers on the other saying they are too difficult to get and should be available on demand. Everyone appears to have forgotten how bad the abortion situation was in this country just a few years ago.

Back in the sixties abortions in Canada could only be legally performed to save the life of the mother and this meant that practically no legal abortions were carried out. But illegal abortions were so commonplace that every physician knew of someone doing them. In Toronto pregnant daughters of the rich automatically were sent to one of the two reliable physicians who did ten to fifteen abortions per week for a cash fee of $500. I well remember attending an annual medical ball in Toronto in 1964 when one of these gentlemen remarked to me, "They pretend they don't know me but I have aborted fifteen of the women in this room." These abortions were done safely with a simple scraping of the womb and the mortality rate was nil.

Unfortunately the service of these physicians were not available to the woman of ordinary means who became pregnant with an unwanted child. Such a woman either had to perform a self-abortion or else turn to one of the backroom "nurse" abortionists who did the job by pumping lysol into the woman's womb. The mortality rate was high and the infection rate ran over 50 per cent and often resulted in lifelong sterility.

By the time I was appointed Chief Coroner I had undergone the unpleasant experience of seeing the bodies of some dozens of young women who had died as the result of these amateur abortions. I was determined to change the abortion laws and decided to organize public pressure to that end. In order to make the public aware of the problem I instructed my coroners to conduct a public inquest into every abortion death and it took only a few of these gruesome stories before the newspapers joined the campaign. The turning point took place on May 14, 1964, following an inquest into the death of Mrs. Lottie Leanne Clarke.

Mrs. Clarke was thirty-four, the mother of three, and had just separated from her husband. She fell in love with twenty-eight-year-old Philip S., a Portuguese immigrant, and after some weeks she discovered that she was pregnant. She confided to a friend that "Philip can't help me and I'll lose my job at the post office if I don't have an abortion."

Mrs. Clarke was told by a friend to visit the home of a woman who was a "practical" nurse at a suburban hospital. The nurse passed a tube into Lottie Clarke's womb and then pumped in a lysol solution. The next day Mrs. Clarke developed severe abdominal cramps with bleeding. She eventually called the police for help and the officer who answered the call sent her to Mount Sinai Hospital by ambulance. At the hospital the admitting physician found her pulse to be 120 and her temperature 103. He immediately began treating her with antibiotics in an attempt to control the infection. Four hours later Mrs. Clarke aborted, passing an eight-week-old foetus. She was placed in a room with three other women who had miscarried and the next day she related her troubles to one of these patients, a Mrs. Rosie Stern. She told how she had scrimped and saved, sometimes going without food, in order to raise the $100 which the abortionist had demanded in advance. Three days later Mrs. Clarke died. The post-mortem showed multiple brain abscesses that had spread from the infection caused by the abortion.

The inquest jury recommended revision of the laws pertaining to therapeutic abortions and this recommendation, following the widespread publicity of Mrs. Clarke's sad death, triggered a whole series of actions. The Toronto *Telegram* started the ball rolling with an editorial "Abortion and the Law," in which they said: "Women continue to die as a result of illegal abortions. Why should doctors operate according to the dictates of their conscience, the mores of the community and still be under a threat of prosecution? Why don't we amend the law to conform with custom? Shouldn't those who are authorities in the field face the problem and come up with constructive answers?"

The Globe and Mail followed with an editorial, "Reforming the Abortion Law," which said it all:

> A study of the incidence of criminal abortions would face our legislators with the fact that Canadian practice in the matter of abortion is not in conformity with Canadian law on the subject and that it is time the two were brought closer together. It has been unofficially estimated that some 75,000 illegal abortions are performed in Canada annually, leaving behind them a trail of dead and maimed women. The jury's recommendation that the law pertaining to therapeutic abortions be revised is also reasonable . . . Dr. Shulman's rider, calling for a federal committee to look at the whole question of abortion and the law was the most valid recommendation to come out of the inquest . . . When society is ready for a reform that legislators refuse to make, the law is placed under a burden which it cannot sustain and it breaks down, bringing all law and all courts into disrespect. The abortion laws are now having this unhealthy effect on Canadian law and courts.

It wasn't only in Toronto that the press reacted. The Belleville *Intelligencer* said, "Dr. Shulman's proposals seem reasonable. Such an amendment to the code would only be permissive—there would be nothing to force any person who objects to abortion for religious reasons to undergo such an operation." The Kingston *Whig-Standard* called for change: "It seems almost unbelievable that, in a society which calls itself enlightened, in the case of conception resulting from rape or incest, abortion is forbidden. Where is the decency and justice in that ignorant view?"

Often the politicians don't listen to the reformers, but this time someone was listening. Guy Favreau, the federal Minister of

Justice, wrote to me on January 27, 1965: "Your recommendation has been carefully noted for consideration in connection with the Criminal Code amendment program." Shortly afterwards the federal government passed a new liberalized abortion law in which they followed exactly the specific recommendations made in 1964 by the coroners' juries.

We fought very hard for these reforms. It is difficult to believe that people today are fighting equally hard to turn the clock back to the bad old days.

11 *The Breathalizer*

Strange though it might seem, only a few years ago the suggestion that drivers be required to take an alcohol breath test on police request was greeted with universal condemnation.

After only a few months as Chief Coroner I realized that I wasn't attacking the major problems. In Toronto a few deaths occurred each year as the result of the depredations of cancer quacks, six or eight from criminal abortions and a handful from drowning, but in 1963 two hundred and fifty-five persons died as the result of car accidents. We routinely did blood alcohol tests on the deceased and found that the number of dead drivers who would have been considered legally impaired was over 50 per cent. On August 25, 1964, I called a press conference to release these figures and called for legislation to bring in the compulsory breathalizer test on police request. Those persons refusing to comply would lose their driver's licence.

Never before had I seen such a solid body of opinion agreeing that I was daft. Lawyer Alan Mintz spoke for the civil liberties association; he condemned such tests as an infringement of civil liberties and said principles involving the presumption of innocence and the right not to testify against oneself were at stake. The provincial Minister of Transport, Irwin Haskett, said that his department was not prepared to consider my suggestions that breath tests be made compulsory: "This is not the solution." *Telegram* columnist Bill Drylie wrote, "Here is Dr. Morton Shulman sticking a shiv into the back of the public. He's asking me to help convict myself if I ever run into a guard rail and the public think I've been into the juice. It's not ruddy likely that I'd help to do that. I'm surprised at the doctor who wants to protect the public so much trying to take away a basic right. Making a breathalizer test mandatory wouldn't cut down on the number of drinking drivers just as the rope has never decreased the number of murders." The three Toronto papers showed a rare unanimity. The *Star* editorialized, "It is a basic concept in law that no person should be compelled to give evidence against himself. Dr. Shulman's suggestion carries too great a risk of erosion of civil liberties for too small a return in convictions." The *Telegram* said, "The repugnant factor in the compulsory breathalizer test is that in effect it requires the suspect to supply evidence against himself. Dr. Shulman . . . has not found the answer." The *Globe* really went overboard: "What evidence does Dr. Shulman have that a breathalizer test is an unerring scientific method of determining whether a suspect driver is drunk, impaired or in good driving order . . . . Dr. Shulman was also somewhat less than scientific in his assessment of the role which liquor plays in traffic fatalities . . . . The breathalizer might (and might not) reduce the traffic casualties but it would make a casualty of justice. One of the basic rules of our system of justice is that a man cannot be compelled to testify against himself. Yet forcing him to take a breathalizer test is forcing him to testify against himself. One can say that the better good of society is served by this contraction of an individual's rights. But can society ever be well served by measures which strike at its foundation? It is encouraging that Attorney General A. A. Wishart does not think so . . . . We do not yet put machines above Magna Carta."

The *Beverage Alcohol Reporter*, organ of the liquor industry, summed it all up in their August 1964 issue — "I would further recommend that Dr. Shulman and other assorted doctors who have been quoting alarming statistics with reference to alcoholism and traffic accidents, check their source of information and also check their own presentation of these statistics so that we cannot challenge them with the old axiom that 'Figures don't lie . . . but liars sure can figure.' "

Fortunately I was more successful with the federal Minister of Justice. I wrote to Mr. Trudeau, who then held that post, pointing out: "If we are to follow the woolly thinking of the Toronto papers we should begin by outlawing fingerprints which compel a person to testify against himself in exactly the same way as does a breathalizer. Surely the forcing of the drinking driver off the road is more important than any right or liberty he may possess to drink, drive and kill." The federal government came to the same conclusion and ultimately brought in the requisite legislation. Today the compulsory breathalizer is law and is taken for granted all across Canada.

Three years later I attempted a second campaign against drinking drivers. In a speech I gave to a consumers group I loudly condemned the provincial government for not having more severe penalties in order to force drinking drivers off the road. As I put it to them, "If someone drinks and drives, take away his driving licence, and if he is subsequently caught driving without a licence, confiscate the vehicle."

The very next day I was stopped a block from my home in a routine police traffic check. The officer asked for and examined my driver's licence and then informed me that it had expired over two years before — apparently my renewal notice from the Department of Transport had been lost in the mail and I had blissfully continued to drive and to break the law. The police officer ordered me from my car and I trudged home and sent my wife back to rescue the car.

I was now grounded and quickly discovered that every driving examiner was booked solid for the next three weeks. Whenever I could I conned my long-suffering wife into driving me about and for the rest of the time I was back to streetcars and taxis. My plight caused considerable amusement among my associates, but I soon learned to enjoy sitting in the back of a car giving driving instructions to Gloria. I took the exam on November 4 and squeaked through but did not tell her about it for another two weeks when she began to show signs of rebellion.

I tried once or twice afterwards to give my "take away their licence" speech but broke up each time and I soon sought other causes to pursue.

12 *Auto Fatalities*

In an effort to cut the number of automobile fatalities I instructed the coroners not only to hold an inquest in each case but also to do a detailed study of each accident so as to determine if the death could have been prevented. It soon became very obvious that there were two factors responsible in addition to the driver: there were structural errors in the automobile itself and defects in highways and road construction.

Because the Coroner's Office was run on a very slim budget and no extra funds were forthcoming from government, I approached the various auto companies to see if any of them would be willing to finance the research which would allow us to hire mechanics after every auto crash to examine the wreckage and see if there had been any structural failures. I also asked each of them to answer a questionnaire relating to their attitude toward enforcement of structural safety minimums through legislation. With the exception of Chrysler, manufacturers and distributors in the country cooperated with this work and Ford sent a cheque for $5,000 to finance it. (Ron Todgham, the president of Chrysler wrote back: "The surprisingly inept wording of the questionnaire sent out by your office strongly brings doubt of both the seriousness and objectivity of the so-called study and virtually precludes response.")

The work on the automobile aspect of highway fatalities proceeded very quickly because we had so much material available in the form of mangled bodies and cars. I soon came to the conclusion that up to one third of highway deaths could have been prevented if cars were built with certain structural changes. By December 27, 1964, our research had progressed sufficiently that I was able to send off the following letter (Ralph Nader published his *Unsafe at any Speed* the following year).

December 27, 1964

Minister of Transport,
Queen's Park
Toronto.

Dear Mr. Haskett,

For sometime I have been disturbed by the increasing toll of highway fatalities in this city and elsewhere. This year there will be an all time high in deaths as a result of auto accidents.

This is one field in which many deaths can be prevented through changes in legislation. Basic responsibility for many of these deaths lies with the auto manufacturers. Drivers cause the accidents but the manufacturers are responsible for the dreadful consequences. They have failed to build cars with a sufficient amount of crashworthiness. 87% of traffic accidents take place at speeds under 40 miles per hour. Well-built cars should be able to withstand crash impact at these relatively low speeds which is why it has been estimated by the Director of Highway Safety Research at Harvard University that crashworthy cars would eliminate 70% of all auto fatalities. I would like to recommend for your consideration that legislation be passed which would make mandatory certain structural minimums for all automobiles sold in Ontario. A very comprehensive group has been drafted by the National Foundation for traffic safety and is currently being considered by several State legislatures. There are 8 basic changes required.

1. Roofs must be noncollapsible with roll over bars like those in racing cars. Doors should be reinforced with beams to protect against side impact. Trunk walls should be able to withstand the impact of objects flying forward after sudden stops.

2. Steering wheels should be collapsible.

3. Interiors should be padded with energy absorbent materials.

4. Shoulder harnesses and neck protectors should be in every car.

5. Cars should have two independent braking systems — emergency brakes should be a true emergency not a parking brake.

6. Obstructions to vision should be removed.

7. Front end surfaces should be rounded. Spikes and spears should be outlawed. Inside knobs should be recessed.

8. Door latches should be strengthened so that they do not fly open on impact.

The Liberty Mutual Insurance Co. of Boston, a pioneer in auto safety, recently incorporated all of these changes in a new automobile and they have estimated that this would add only $10.00 to cost of manufacturing the car.

The terrible slaughter on the Highways of North America cannot continue. Sooner or later steps must be taken to cut the death toll. If Ontario leads in these changes she will be responsible for a revolution in car habits that will save thousands of lives yearly.

Please excuse my presumption in writing to you on this matter; however it is a matter of the greatest importance to my office and one in which I believe many lives could be saved.

The Minister of Transport gave my letter a polite acknowledgement and then forgot the whole affair. But in Ottawa C. M. Drury, the Minister of Industry, was intrigued by the press reports and invited me to join a federally sponsored Committee on Traffic Safety which he was then setting up. The committee consisted of representatives of each provincial Minister of Transport and several federal transport officials plus one member of Parliament and myself. We met about half a dozen times over the next two years and formulated a series of safety standards which largely followed the requests in my original letter to Irwin Haskett.

In June 1965 the Ford Motor Company invited me to visit Dearborn, Michigan, to go through their plant; they wanted to hear my suggestions about improving auto safety and they also wanted to show me what they were doing themselves. I spent two days at the company's safety research laboratory and then went off to Detroit where General Motors gave me a similar tour. I came back convinced that one aspect of auto accidents was being completely ignored — that of roadside hazards.

General Motors had given me a study done at Cornell University called "Automotive Crash Injury Research Program" which illustrated the right and wrong ways to build a highway. As I drove around Toronto I found that our highways and expressways could have been used as Cornell's models for the wrong ways — we had quite literally done everything wrong. I now went back through our statistics to see how many deaths had taken place as a result of autos striking improperly placed roadside obstructions and found that there had been several every month. Seeing that every highway had been built incorrectly I decided to concentrate on our newest local highway, Metropolitan Toronto's Don Valley Parkway. I found that four people had died and eighty-six had been injured in one hundred and thirty-nine accidents from January to May on the eight miles of this brand new expressway. The engineers had made every mistake in the book.

They had placed the light standards in front of the guard rails instead of behind them. They had used concrete light standards instead of collapsible aluminum ones. They had dug steep slopes beside unguarded highway. They had failed to place guard rails to protect concrete bridge supports and abutments. They had not bothered to curve the guard rail ends to prevent automobiles being skewered.

I spent one Sunday afternoon on the parkway taking pictures of all these errors and on August 16, 1965, issued an "Action Report" illustrating every mistake and saying that basic safety essentials had been ignored. I called for massive changes in the expressway so as to prevent unnecessary deaths.

Metro Traffic Commissioner Sam Cass responded immediately, denying that the Don Valley was badly built and saying that changes were unlikely. He also pointed out that his department did not have unlimited funds to make changes and that many of the things I was suggesting had not been known when the parkway was built. He concluded that the parkway had "a surprisingly good" safety record.

As if to punctuate my report the very next day forty-five-year-old Mary Greenan was instantly killed when her car struck a concrete post on the parkway. Metro Chairman William Allen now ordered Sam Cass to prepare a detailed safety study of the parkway.

On September 3, Traffic Commissioner Cass and Road Commissioner George Grant presented their safety studies to Mr. Allen. They accused me of exaggeration and said they did not have either the facilities or the money to go "chasing phantoms" of unproven safety proposals. They maintained that the Don Valley was one of the safest super roads in North America. Mr. Cass said that highway poles must be strong enough to withstand high wind velocity and that the light-weight standards that I had recommended would break off on impact and send "a deadly missile" into the path of other motorists. Referring to the guard rails, Commissioner Grant said intensive research by traffic experts had shown that rails can cause as many or more hazards then they prevent. He said the rails have a tendency to force a straying vehicle back onto the road out of control where it causes a multiple accident. As for protecting motorists from the light poles, Mr. Cass said accident records proved cars can receive as much damage from hitting the rail itself. Mr. Grant said it would be possible to curve the ends of guard rails away from the road to prevent cars being speared by them but this would eliminate the chance a motorist now had to miss the rail by going behind it!

I replied to their arguments by pointing out that there was an average of 114.1 accidents per 100 million miles on U.S. four-lane highways while the Don Valley figure was 162.2. The U.S. personal accident rate was 36.2 while the parkway had a rate of 86.4. The Metro Transportation Committee now invited me to appear before them with Mr. Cass so that they could consider the matter. The committee was not unanimous in wanting to hear me. Etobicoke Reeve John MacBeth opposed the invitation: "He's not the expert he thinks he is. He's not an expert in highway safety and I'm not prepared to listen to him. He just has no knowledge of what he is talking about." Committee chairman Scarboro Reeve Albert Campbell wondered "whether Dr. Shulman would like Metro traffic experts telling him how to do an appendectomy," and Metro Chairman William Allen said it was the drivers' own fault if they smashed themselves up while speeding.

The meeting itself was a chilly one. I urged the city fathers to invite the prestigious Traffic Institute of Northwestern University to come to Toronto and make a study of the city's traffic situation. They wanted none of that and voted it down unanimously. They then flatly rejected all the charges that the Don Valley Parkway was unsafe and poorly designed.

Several months later, in May 1966, a police constable came to my home one evening and left me a parcel containing a secret traffic survey done in Toronto by the National Safety Council in 1960. The officer said that the report had been commissioned by the police but that senior officials had been very unhappy at the results and had ordered it not made public and that it had sat buried in police files for the previous five years.

There was indeed good reason for the report to be suppressed; it contained an exhaustive survey of every aspect of Toronto traffic control ranging from accident rates to traffic engineering to police traffic courts and in not one category did Toronto fulfill even the minimum standards. In fact, in six of the eight categories the city had only between 53 and 73 per cent of the minimum requirements. Worse, the Safety Council had made a series of recommendations in each category to enable the city to come up to standards and all of these had been ignored.

I released the report at once and flayed the civil officials who had suppressed and ignored it. This did not enhance my popularity at City Hall but because the figures had been prepared not by me but by the National Safety Council my critics found themselves in the uncomfortable position of having to attack the accuracy of the National Safety Council. They did their best.

Chairman of the Metro Police Commission, Magistrate C. O. Bick was quoted in the Press as saying, "We didn't feel it was a proper analysis. Their analyses and appraisals of situations were based too much on experiences of the United States." Metro Traffic Commissioner Sam Cass said that, "If there is anything

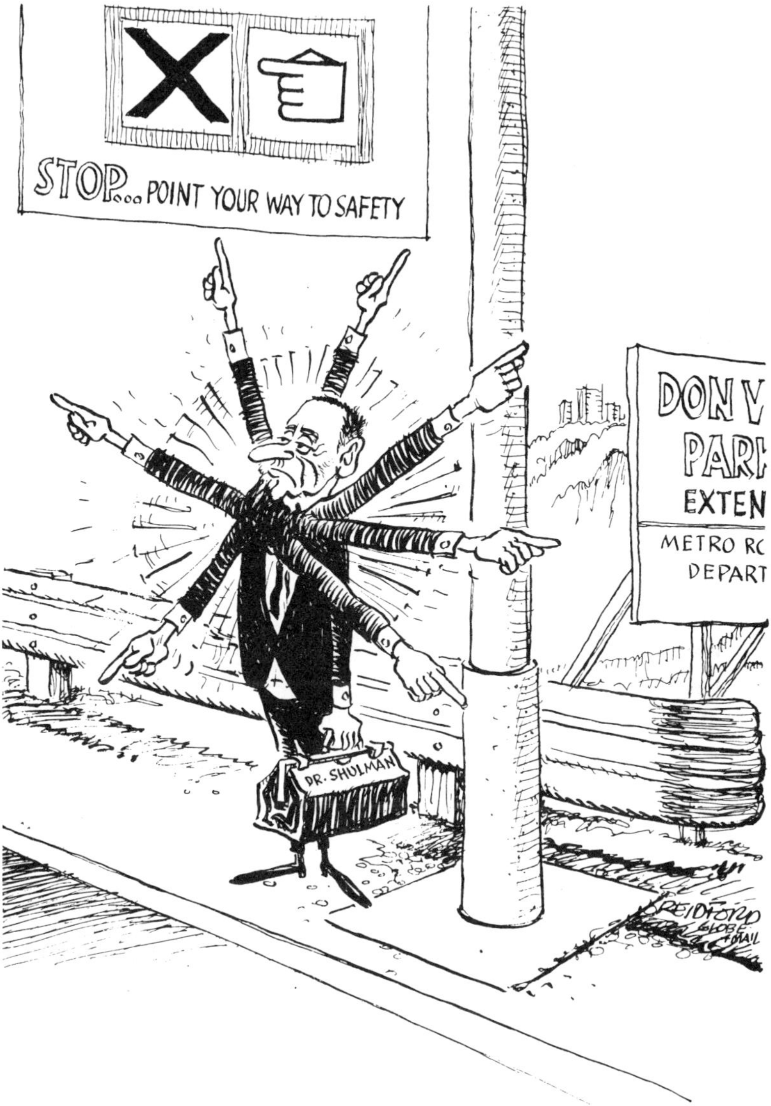
STOP... POINT YOUR WAY TO SAFETY
DON V
PARK
EXTEN
METRO RO
DEPART
DR. SHULMAN
REIDFORD
GLOBE
+ MAIL

wrong with Metro's traffic control and supervision methods it has not been shown up. We are still one of the safest cities in North America. That belies any phony statistical analysis that anyone can come up with."

Other officials took refuge in faulty memory. The *Toronto Star* phoned the National Safety Council to ask who had ordered the study and they informed the paper that the request had come from Toronto's Deputy Chief of Police. But the Deputy said, "I don't recall any survey. I don't know anything about it." Metro Chairman William Allen said, "I know of no survey. I have no idea what Dr. Shulman is talking about and furthermore I don't care." Fred Gardiner who had been Metro Chairman in 1960 said, "The National Safety Council was never engaged by us to do it and no recommendations were received so far as I know."

In light of all the confusion, and encouraged both by letters and phone calls from the public and by editorials in all the newspapers, I decided to put together an overall action program to reduce Toronto's traffic toll. I released my ten-point program in June 1966 and called for:

- Compulsory annual auto inspection to force drivers to keep their cars in safe condition
- Compulsory driving instruction in high schools
- Installation of guard rails along the sidewalk on main downtown streets to stop pedestrians crossing except at lights and crosswalks
- Guard rails in the middle of expressways
- Replacement of concrete poles with aluminum ones
- More traffic police
- More one-way streets
- Replacement of police by crown attorneys in traffic courts

I am sorry to say that I largely failed in my efforts to institute this program. Guard rails were put on the expressways and aluminum poles have gradually replaced concrete ones, but the bulk of the "Action Program" of 1966 never received any action.

13 *My Second Firing — 1965*

One of the major deficiencies at the Metro Coroner's Office was the fact that no one had ever assembled and collected statistics on the various deaths being investigated. I determined to change this situation and immediately after my appointment began the collection and categorization of information on each death. Beginning in February 1964 the Coroner's Office published an annual report showing all the information collected in the previous year and making various recommendations to reduce deaths in coming years. To say that my report was not acclaimed by the provincial government is an understatement of gross proportions. My second report came close to being my last (I published four before they finally fired me).

The 1963 report was a slim volume of twenty-four pages consisting almost entirely of statistical data with the only editorial comment coming on the final page. "1963 was a year of reorganization in which a small efficient staff was hired, proper reporting of deaths was begun, policing of cremations was enforced and work was distributed by area to the eighteen coroners on staff. The philosophy that the prime function of the Coroner's Office was to prevent deaths was expounded and has produced a significant change in the activities of this office."

The 1964 report was a more ambitious document; fifty-four pages long, it contained extensive statistical data on the causes of Toronto deaths, but also included an analysis of the important inquests of the year including the George, Power and Shouldice cases, a breakdown of the auto deaths with suggestions for changes in auto construction, a lengthy write-up on the benefits of the breathalizer test and it finished up by saying: "In summary, while 1963 was a year of reorganization, 1964 was a year of achievement. Progress was made in the fields of safety, in construction and medicine. The first positive results have come from our collaboration in research. Recommendations were made in the fields of automobile safety, the drinking driver, criminal abortion and the medical incompetent. It is our hope that 1965 will see the carrying out of at least some of these recommendations with consequent lowering of mortality in these fields."

Looking back I see that the report was unnecessarily critical of the slowness of the Attorney General's department in making reforms and I certainly used bad judgment in tweaking their noses over their failure to act against a drunken coroner whom I finally suspended when they refused to do so. Perhaps most seriously, I had heavily criticized the College of Physicians and Surgeons for their failure to act against cancer quacks and suggested that a public representative be appointed to their discipline committee.

I was not unaware of the controversial nature of the report and decided to avoid trouble by submitting it first to the Attorney General. There now was a new Attorney General, Arthur Wishart, with whom to contend. In manner he was the typical country lawyer. Modest, self-effacing, and tenacious, he inspired an uncommon loyalty in his staff. On February 10, 1965, I left a copy of my report with his deputy and asked him to advise me of any corrections or deletions which they wished me to make. I said that I planned to send it to the printer on March 1, and to please advise me before that date. I did not hear back from the Attorney General or his staff and so printed the report and released it to the public on March 31, 1965. The reaction was not slow in appearing.

The very next day the *Telegram* ran a front-page story headlined "Shulman to be Fired" and beginning, "The dismissal of Metro's fiery Chief Coroner Dr. Morton Shulman is imminent. . . . Attorney General Arthur Wishart, thoroughly exasperated by the latest criticisms of his department and staff by the boat-rocking Dr. Shulman, wants to abolish the post of Chief Coroner . . . an almost identical attempt to get rid of Dr. Shulman a year ago ended in crushing failure for the department and for the then Attorney General Fred Cass." The *Telegram* accompanied their article with an editorial calling me "ham-fisted" and saying, "Dr. Shulman went beyond good judgment when he suggested that a layman should be appointed to the disciplinary committee of the Ontario College of Physicians . . . no layman possesses the professional qualifications to determine the degree of fault by a doctor." (Seven years later the government finally did appoint the first lay member to the disciplinary committee.)

Dr. Cotnam fired the next salvo and the next day's papers carried a front-page story headlined, "Shulman a swell head says Cotnam." The article began: "Metro Chief Coroner Morton Shulman is inflated by the idea of his own importance, Ontario Supervising Coroner H. B. Cotnam told the *Telegram* yesterday. Dr. Cotnam delivered a broadside in which he charged that part of Dr. Shulman's report is a mixture of truth and half truths. . . . Dr. Cotnam poured scorn on Dr. Shulman's suggestion for a public watchdog on the Ontario College of Physicians and Surgeons' Discipline Committee. 'This would be like putting a mechanic on the Dental Discipline Committee or letting an ice cream vendor assess the actions of lawyers!'"

Attorney General Arthur Wishart contributed that it was an impossible situation when an official of his department tells him publicly how to run it. "I shall shortly decide on what action will be taken." He did not say whether he intended to fire me from my $9,000-a-year post, but he left no doubt that I "was in for more than a wrist slapping."

I was astounded at all of this because I had given the Attorney General the report weeks before, asking for suggestions and none had been forthcoming; now the roof appeared to be falling in. I demanded (and got) a meeting with John Robarts in order to present my side of it. I met the Premier in his office on April 3, was greeted warmly and he listened sympathetically to my tale of woe. He was noncommittal about my future but said he would discuss it with Attorney General Wishart.

Meanwhile I received an outpouring of support from press and public. Strangely enough, it was led by the *Telegram* who com-

'DR. SHULMAN IS NOT RESPONDING TO TREATMENT'

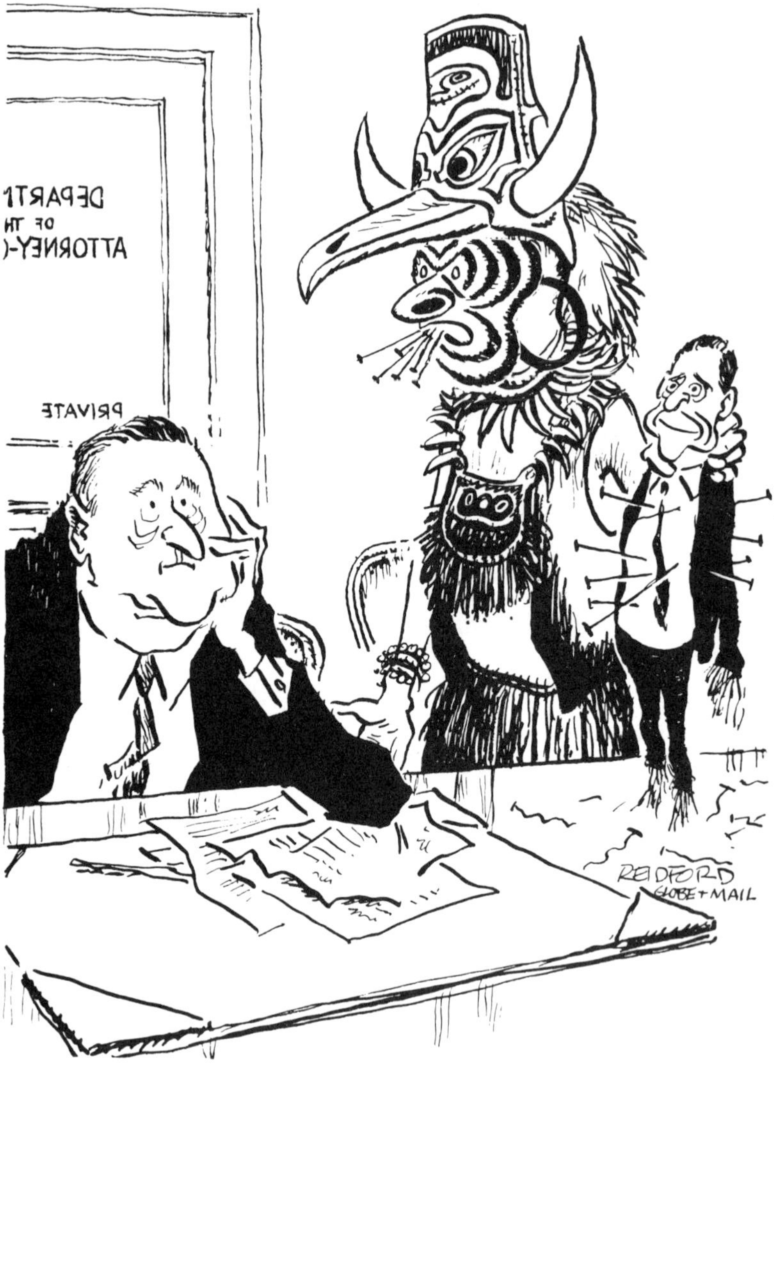

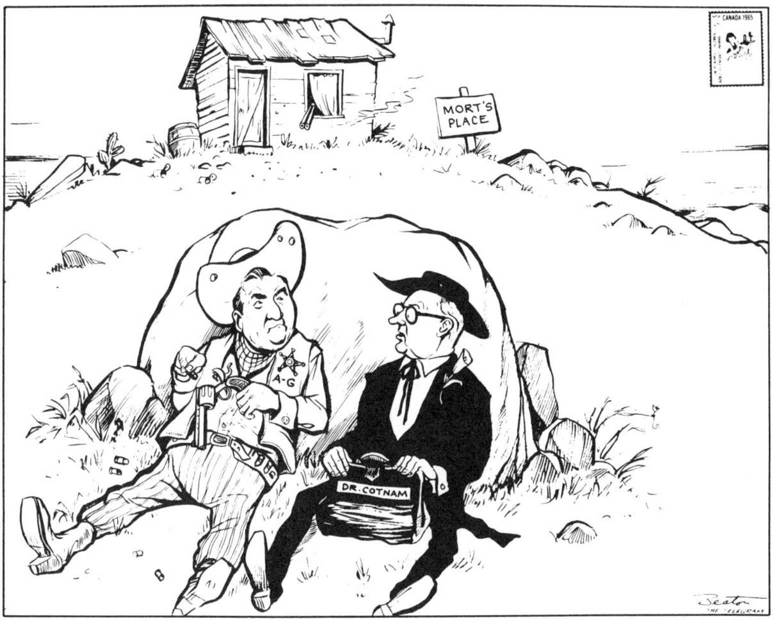

"GO IN THAR 'N GET HIM, PARDNER."

pletely reversed their editorial of April 1, and on April 2 wrote: "Dr. Shulman is doing his job as he sees it and the public generally will see it the same way." The *Globe* was very flattering. "As a result of Dr. Shulman's activities it is safer for people to go to work in this town, safer for them to go to hospital, safer even for them to go to jail. But his work is not finished. It will never be finished. So long as there are negligent, incompetent and crooked people with the lives of other people in their hands (and such are always with us) there will be a need for Dr. Shulman." The *Star* presented my arguments in detail."As his authority for taking such a hefty swipe at the Establishment, Dr. Shulman cites a sentence in *Coroners' Practice*, 'the coroner is an entirely independent functionary who is answerable to no one save the public and represents no other interest' . . .the public will continue to applaud his efforts to explore every possible cause of mysterious death — at whatever cost to the A.G.'s nerves."

This furore was not quite as mysterious as it appeared to me at the time. *Telegram* reporter Peter Bruton dug into the story and discovered that after the A.G.'s officials had read the report in February they had had numerous criticisms and objections but did not voice them to me for fear that at some later date I might accuse them of gagging me. The same officials deliberately planted the story with the *Telegram* that I was to be fired with the idea of putting sufficient pressure on me to make me come to heel. As Bruton put it, "The government source insisted that Dr. Shulman not receive advance warning of the *Tely* story. Surprise and shock were key factors in the government's strategy. Dr. Shulman is a maverick and it is doubtful whether he can remain knuckled under for any period of time. But the government is apparently well satisfied that it has won this round."

After this incident I received a phoned invitation to lunch with Dalton Bales and Hugh Latimer, and Bales advised me: "Mr. Wishart is very busy, so we would rather you didn't bother him with any further troubles in your department. If there is any difficulty, please call me directly and I will straighten it out."

A new happier relationship with the Tory government bloomed in the most extraordinary way. Just days after the government had said they were going to fire me the former Attorney General and now Minister of Lands and Forests, Kelso Roberts, had risen on April 6 at the sixteenth anniversary meeting of the Spadina Conservatives Women's Club to praise my "crusading spirit" and to suggest that I be asked to run as the Conservative candidate in the forthcoming federal by-election in Spadina riding. Mr. Roberts said, "Dr. Shulman has shown a great deal of interest in the welfare of people and I can confidently state that a person so disposed would have a far wider field of activity as a federal member of Parliament than in any capacity of a more local nature that I could think of."

Tories had been suggesting many places I should go, but this was the first one to suggest Ottawa. I replied that I was amazed and flattered but not interested: "I have no intention now or in the future of ever running for any political office."

I had barely got over that shock when I started getting phone calls from various party functionaries asking if I would take the Conservative nomination in the provincial riding of Bracondale.

The sitting member had died and a by-election was about to be called. I didn't give their offer serious consideration and was amused when hints began to appear in the press in late May that the Tory party needed me. One Tory official was quoted as saying, "There is no question that Morton Shulman would be a great asset on the Conservative benches and would make a fine contribution to legislative debate."

Left unsaid was the little matter that if I agreed to run I would have to resign my post as Chief Coroner, and, to boot, the seat of Bracondale was due to disappear in the next provincial redistribution. I was suspicious of the Tories' intentions and decided that this was just a more subtle way to get rid of me. I declined their kind offer with thanks, saying "I do not wish to be an MPP — I shall never run for provincial parliament or any other elected post — I am not a politician."

14 *General Improvements*

Meanwhile I had been active on other fronts. It had been obvious to me for many years that the way coroners' inquests were run was on occasion grossly unjust to persons involved. If a person were believed to be responsible for conditions leading to someone else's death he would often be badgered and harassed by both the coroner and the Crown Attorney, sometimes quite unfairly. I felt that any person in such a position should be entitled to the advice and aid of his own lawyer, but the Coroner's Act said that this was allowed only at the whim of the coroner, and for over twenty years coroners had rarely granted this privilege.

After my appointment as Chief Coroner I began to extend this privilege at all the inquests I conducted personally and on April 28, 1965, I appeared before Chief Justice McRuer, who was then conducting his Royal Commission on Human Rights, to suggest that the Coroner's Act should be amended to allow the lawyers of affected persons to ask questions as a right rather than a privilege.

A parallel problem was the lack of cooperation from the Crown Attorney's Office in providing legal counsel for the coroner. None of the coroners had legal training and this meant that we had to rely on the Crown Attorney for advice. But crown attorneys only attended those inquests which they considered important, so in order to ensure a minimum of legal difficulties I began to write the Crown Attorney asking him to send a representative for cases that might involve complications. This was often refused, as the following exchange of letters indicates:

April 5, 1965.

To The Crown Attorney
Re: Inquest on James A. Heath, deceased.
Dear Sirs: Due to the unusual circumstances in the above mentioned case, I would like a crown.attorney to be present at the inquest which will be held at 86 Lombard Street, April 15, 1965, at 7:30 p.m.

Dr. M.P. Shulman

April 6, 1965.

Re: Inquest on James A. Heath, deceased.
Dear Sir: I saw no unusual circumstances set out in your statement upon issuing your warrant and do not propose to assign a Crown Attorney to this inquest.

Yours truly,
Mr. Langdon,
Deputy Crown Attorney.

April 9, 1965.

To The Crown Attorney
Re: Inquest on James A. Heath, deceased.
As there may be legal questions as to whether certain evidence is admissible in this particular inquest I would again request the attendance of a representative of the Crown.

M. Shulman.

April 12, 1965.

Morton Shulman, Chief Coroner
Dear Sir:
Re: Inquest James Heath, deceased.
Would you please outline the evidence to which you refer in your letter of April 9th.

Mr. Langdon.

April 14, 1965.

Mr. Langdon
Dear Mr. Langdon:
The evidence to which I refer is the confusion and long delay incidental in sending rescue vehicles to the scene of this accident.

M. Shulman.

April 18, 1965.

M. Shulman:
Your letter of April 14th has just now reached me. The evidence outlined in this letter does not seem to me to involve any question of admissibility which would necessitate the attendence of an Assistant Crown Attorney.

Mr. Langdon

In May 1965 I decided to widen the number of inquests in which lawyers participated and so I issued instructions that beginning August 1, 1965, every coroner under my jurisdiction was to permit lawyers to participate as counsel in inquests. To my great delight Supervising Coroner H. B. Cotnam agreed with me, saying "I see nothing wrong with the principle. It's a democratic prerogative. At one time I felt that extending this privilege to lawyers would turn inquests into a shambles and make them marathons. I thought that way because that was the way I had been conditioned to think but experience has made me change my mind."

And it took a long time, but in 1972 the provincial government brought in an amendment to the Coroner's Act giving affected persons at an inquest the right to cross examine either in person or through their counsel.

I had been surprised at Dr. Cotnam's generous comments about the appearance of lawyers at inquests and responded in kind. This ushered in a period of relative calm at the morgue with no public battles between the Attorney General's department and myself.

For over a generation a coroner's appointment was a matter of minor patronage given out at the request and with the approval of the local Tory MPP. Although the appointment was a minor matter to the politicians concerned, it was of major importance to a doctor seeking a coronership because of the prestige, the income and the entry to hospitals; as a result there were tremendous pressures exerted to get such appointments.

After I became Chief Coroner I was very conscious of the problem of these appointments and attempted to persuade the government to make them on a more rational basis. One case in particular pointed up the foolish way things were then carried out — an eighty-three-year old Toronto physician was appointed to the post though he was already so senile that he could not write out his reports. I suggested that in future coroners' appointments be made only when a vacancy required an appointment and then only after public advertisement and on a basis of merit. The government didn't think much of that idea and nothing came of it.

In March 1966 the only coroner of the eighteen on staff who lived in North Toronto retired and I inquired at various hospitals and at the university for a successor to him. Dr. George Sereny was highly recommended to me as a specialist in internal medicine and as a scientist, and as I had already met him socially and been favourably impressed I wrote to Dr. Cotnam on March 23, recommending his appointment. Several months passed with no action and in June I phoned Dr. Cotnam to find out what was the problem. Dr. Cotnam said that he did not know and that he had forwarded all the information to Frank Wilson, the Deputy Assistant Attorney General. On June 7, 1966, I phoned Wilson to inquire and my secretary transcribed the conversations as follows.

Myself: Frank, I am calling you about the appointment of George Sereny as a coroner in North York. Dr. Cotnam says he forwarded all the facts to you.

Wilson: What is his name?

Myself: Sereny.

Wilson: How do you spell it?

Myself: S-E-R-E-N-Y. He is very highly qualified.

Wilson: What is his nationality?

Myself: He is a Canadian citizen who was born in Hungary and came here after the war.

Wilson: Where does he live—in West Toronto?
Myself: No, he lives in North Toronto, where we need the coroner.
Wilson: Don't they all live in West Toronto?
Myself: Now, Frank, that went out in Germany in 1945.
Wilson: Well, some persons' applications take much longer to process than others.
Myself: His application has been in for a long time now and I would certainly appreciate your putting it through.
Wilson: Well, we will see.

Dr. Sereny never heard from the Attorney General's office and he did not receive his appointment. However, a few months later the Attorney General did appoint two new coroners in Toronto, Dr. Ross Cameron Bennett and Dr. Cranston.

Both of these gentlemen were undoubtedly very fine doctors but they both resided in east Toronto where we already had a surplus of coroners. No one was appointed to service the north end of the city. By now I was convinced that the Attorney General's office was run by some perverse child, determined to do the wrong thing. I suspect that they reciprocated my feelings.

Cremations were a constant worry and anxiety during my years at the Coroner's Office and they kept me in continual hot water with my superiors.

My concern started back in 1961 (when I was still an assistant coroner) with a case of murder in the United States which was confessed to but in which no post-mortem could be performed because the body had been cremated. This sparked my interest and I took a close look at the Ontario procedure. I found it pretty sloppy — before a cremation could be carried out a coroner was required to sign a certificate of permission, but these were being signed holus-bolus and in many cases with absolutely no investigation being carried out. I wrote the Attorney General's office at the time and recommended numerous reforms but nothing came of my suggestions.

In March 1963, immediately after my appointment, I made radical changes in the reporting and investigation of these cases and I insisted that an investigation take place in every case. I was, however, still worried that the odd murder might slip through. So on March 27, 1963, I wrote to Dr. Cotnam to suggest that in future "all cases requesting cremation, which have not been treated in hospital with a definite diagnosis established, require the performance of a post-mortem before cremation." Dr. Cotnam wrote back to me on April 3, 1963, saying, "I will forward your recommendation to the proper authorities as you have requested although my opinion in this matter does not coincide with yours."

I did not learn until many years later that the letter Dr. Cotnam sent to the Attorney General on April 3 somewhat altered my proposal. He wrote that I had suggested "*All* bodies for cremation be sent for complete medico-legal autopsies prior to cremation regardless of whether they die in hospital or not and without any consideration of the circumstances surrounding these deaths." His letter continued: "I knew, Sir, that we could expect some thoughtless and ill-conceived proposal from Dr. Shulman but I never dreamed of one so far left of centre, as it were." Dr. Cotnam wrote this letter only three weeks after I had begun my job—but fortunately for my equanimity I was completely unaware of it.

Although it was of no practical value I did feel gratified to receive the moral support of the province's crime lab on this issue. On June 6, 1963, its director, Dr. H. Ward Smith, learned of the controversy and wrote to me, "I have not written on this topic of the necessity of post-mortems before cremation. I did not think it was necessary to do so. I cannot see any circumstances where a post-mortem would not be required if a cremation is contemplated."

As the years passed I continued to argue with the Attorney General's department over cremations but I made absolutely no progress. One of my constant aggravations was over the sheer waste of money involved. A coroner was sent to investigate every cremation, but 25 per cent of all of these deaths had already been investigated by the same or another coroner because the death had fallen under one of the categories reportable under the Coroner's Act. It just didn't make any sense to me to repeat all these investigations, nor did it make any sense to put the bereaved family to the unnecessary expense of paying for their certificates.

On May 11, 1966, I was still trying. I wrote to Attorney General

Wishart on that date: "Over 25 per cent of the calls on which we are sending coroners to sign cremation certificates are duplications of calls which coroners have already investigated. We certainly want every suspicious case investigated, but a great deal of money could be saved by eliminating the duplications and the unnecessary investigations of normal deaths." I did not receive any reply from Mr. Wishart but a few days later his Assistant Deputy Frank Wilson phoned me with this gem, "You are aware of course that cremation fees are not paid out of public funds, so we are not wasting public funds, we are wasting the public's funds." (Cremation fees are not paid out of the treasury, so he was technically quite correct.)

As late as February 7, 1967, I met Mr. Wishart himself and raised this matter with him. He replied that the amount of money involved was really not very much but he would take a look at it.

It is depressing to note that the same duplication and waste still goes on today. Every year since 1967 a private member's bill has been introduced in the Ontario legislature to eliminate this foolishness but the succession of Attorneys General and Solicitors General who have followed Arthur Wishart have all been equally unimpressed.

For me the most satisfying change I made as Chief Coroner was to open up the coroners' autopsy room to research scientists. Some medical research can only be carried out on parts of the bodies of recently dead persons: likewise, successful organ transplants require healthy organs from the recently dead. As a rule the autopsies that take place in general hospitals are of little help for they normally take place after a lengthy illness and the body organs are often badly shrivelled or diseased.

What are needed are healthy organs from the bodies of accident victims and these are available only at a coroner's autopsy. Shortly after I received my appointment as Chief Coroner, we had a form printed which gave permission for such research and after every death we routinely asked the next of kin to sign permission for use of the deceased's organs. No one ever refused and we soon had a bevy of research scientists depending upon us.

The Attorney General's department did not approve and on

October 6, 1964, I received a letter from Dr. Cotnam ordering me to restrict attendance at autopsies to the Chief Coroner's staff. I appealed over his head to Assistant Deputy Attorney General Frank Wilson who wrote to me saying I had no legal right to carry on this type of work. He did not, however, expressly forbid my carrying it on and in view of his indecision and the great results we were getting I just went ahead and hoped for the best. The results were spectacular.

The first project was begun by a research team from the Banting Institute headed by Dr. Calvin Ezrin who made a study of the pituitary glands supplied from our autopsies. On December 11, 1964, Dr. Ezrin announced that his team had made a major contribution to medical knowledge of the human pituitary gland as a result of this work. He announced: "My co-workers and I have discovered that the pituitary gland is composed of 7 types of cells not just 2 as was previously believed. We have cracked the code of the pituitary gland—each different type of cell secretes a different hormone. The findings will be of significance in treating breast cancer and in the prevention of blindness in certain diabetic patients. This morgue work has confirmed what previously had been only suspicions."

Dr. Ezrin's public announcement brought in a flood of requests from other researchers and we soon had a dozen different projects underway. The department of psychiatry at the University of Toronto was supplied with pineal glands for research into their role in psychiatric illness. The department of orthopedic surgery at the Toronto General Hospital was supplied with lumbar discs in order to study the possibility of dissolving ruptured discs with a drug called chymopapin. This worked beautifully and led to a completely new non-surgical treatment of back disc disease. I took special pleasure from this discovery because as a result of it one of my closest friends was able to avoid a major operation on his spine. The Banting Institute was supplied with heart valves for research into the possibility of transplanting them into living humans suffering from heart disease. The department of biochemistry at the University of Toronto was supplied with kidneys for their study of kidney enzymes. Of immediate value was the supplying of kidneys to the Toronto Western Hospital who successfully used them for human transplants. Possibly most important of all was the work done by Dr. W. S. Hartroft at the Hospital for Sick Children. We supplied him with heart muscles from cadavers for his work on the basic causes of heart disease.

Unfortunately, after my dismissal in 1967 all co-operation with medical research was stopped on the grounds of legal uncertainty. This has been my greatest regret about losing my job.

15 *How to Become an Author*

On the same day in February, 1966 I received two delegations at my office—one from McGraw-Hill, the book publishers, and the other from the CBC.

The two gentlemen from McGraw-Hill introduced themselves as Vice President Lorne Wilkinson and trade editor Ron Hume. They explained that McGraw-Hill had set up its Canadian branch too late to pick up any established authors and they were beating the bushes looking for "names" who might write books for them. They had heard of my good fortune in the financial markets and had come to ask me to write a book on the subject. This sounded like a great idea, but I had never written anything longer than a letter before this and was not sure what was involved. My doubts were quickly settled when my two visitors offered to pay me a $10,000 advance for a finished manuscript. They asked me when I thought it could be ready and I asked them if four weeks would be alright. They stared in disbelief and assured me that would be fine.

Spurred on by the $10,000 prize my secretary and I turned out the book in exactly three weeks; I wrote a chapter each night at home in longhand and Ann typed it the next night after our medical work was done. I gave her the choice of being paid overtime or taking a 10 per cent interest of the book. She took the 10 per cent, as a result of which she ultimately received $26,000 for her typing effort.

We needed a title for the book and, try as we might, couldn't think of anything suitable. Finally I laughingly said, "Put down *Anyone Can Make A Million* — it will do until we find a proper title."

The officials at McGraw-Hill were pleasantly surprised at the rapid delivery and modestly pleased at the contents; they decided on an October publication date and optimistically printed 3,500 copies. We never could think of a good title for the book and finally it went to print carrying its original temporary one.

Canada is not a good book country and a sale of 5,000 is considered a bestseller. As a result almost no one in this country can make a living writing books (Pierre Berton is the one big exception and perhaps Farley Mowat). My $10,000 advance was a record up to that time and was given by McGraw-Hill only because of their desperate need for authors. They had no hope of breaking even on their investment.

The book sold reasonably well, helped considerably by the sale of serial rights to *Weekend* magazine. By Christmas McGraw-Hill was very happy to have sold their 3,500 books and they now ordered another 3,500. I was ecstatic at my literary success.

I was now summoned to the New York headquarters of McGraw-Hill where I was taken to lunch by a pretty young junior editor who told me the company was going to publish the U.S. edition in March and had decided to make an initial printing of 2,500. I didn't think that was very many and the young lady informed me that the great Harold McGraw himself had read my book and had decided it was similar to a dozen that had preceded it and would never sell. He hadn't wanted to publish the book at all and was only proceeding because my contract required that a U.S. edition be published. I returned to Toronto somewhat subdued.

The whole secret of selling a book is to let the public know that the book is available, but because paid advertising is uneconomic the only avenue open to this end is to get on radio or TV shows or to receive newspaper reviews. McGraw-Hill had no hope of success for *Anyone* in the U.S. and so made no effort to get me on TV. However, my young editor felt sorry for me and in order to show me that McGraw-Hill really cared she booked me on to a radio show emanating from New York — the Long John Nebel show. I asked her if she thought it was worth coming to New York just to do one radio show and she assured me that Long John had a very large listening audience. I was told to take the afternoon plane (economy class please) and to come to the McGraw-Hill office. When I arrived my editor told me what she had somehow forgotten to mention before—that Long John's show went on the air at 12:30 A.M. and continued until 5:30 in the morning. To counter my dismay she then took me over to Brentano's main book store where I viewed their front window filled with my books. I would have been more impressed if my friend Marika Robert had not told me of her New York experience with her first novel. Her publisher took her to half a dozen book stores and each one featured her book in the window. The next day she returned to the stores to show off to her husband but the books had disappeared from every window. Apparently it is standard practice in New York to give authors from the boondocks a phony one-hour tour during which the stores oblige by displaying the book.

That night I appeared on the Long John Nebel show and found it different from any other radio show I had ever heard. Long John had brought in two experts to "discuss" my book with me, Bob Metz, the stock market critic from the *New York Times* and Art Lottman, a life insurance expert, and for five hours these two gentlemen cut me into little pieces. They didn't approve of anything I had written and took it as an act of ultimate impudence for a doctor from Canada to come to the big city and give "them" advice on the stock market. They were merciless and I was no match for them. By 4:00 A.M. tempers had risen so high that over some minor point Lottman and I jumped to our feet and were screaming at each other, only to be interrupted by Long John crying "Commercial time — Stay right where you are and we'll start again at this point in just 60 seconds." It was too much. I dissolved into giggles and was unable to restore my equilibrium for the balance of the show. At 5:30 I staggered from the studio and returned to my hotel feeling about two inches high.

At noon my wife Gloria pulled me from bed to return to Toronto but before heading for the airport I insisted that we go to Brentano's. Sure enough, my book had disappeared from the window, and worse, we found that it was also gone from the store's shelves. I was completely dejected and started out of the store but Gloria had heard Marika's story and demanded that I complain to the manager. I was too embarrassed to do so and Gloria said, "Well, I will then," and marched up to Brentano's office. She returned a few minutes later to announce with amazement, "They sold every copy this morning."

From then on it was clear sailing. Johnny Carson had been unable to sleep that night and had tuned in to Long John Nebel and had been amused. The next day he invited me to come on his show and soon Merv Griffen and the other big shows followed suit. The book sold out everywhere and jumped on to the *New York Times* bestseller list where it stayed for thirty weeks and for one glorious week was the U.S. number one bestseller.

I'm not sure what in particular in the book caused this surprising success—I had excoriated the average man's investments in stocks, bonds, life insurance, mortgages and bank savings because of inflation and had suggested the purchase of tangibles, especially gold. This produced a great response from the book-buying public but the financial page reviewers thought I was off my nut. I take some pleasure in looking back at their comments.

Harry Halliwell, the financial editor of the *Telegram* wrote:

> A favourite question directed to this department has been "Is Shulman Right . . . Should I buy gold in expectation of a price rise to $70.00 an ounce or even more?" My answer usually runs along these lines. "In my view the Americans are the most astute business men in the world. They have allowed billions of dollars' worth of gold to leave their country in recent years at $35.00 an ounce. Will they buy it back at $70.00? To me it just doesn't add up". Most of the debate and speculation about the price of gold centres on false assumptions, outmoded economic theories and wishful thinking. Among the false assumptions, the worst is that persistent U.S. balance of payments difficulties are evidence that the U.S. dollar is weak—which is utter nonsense.

Alistair Dow wrote in the *Monetary Times:* "Shulman has an unfortunate tendency to preach his own conviction, based apparently on very shallow reasoning, that the price of gold is bound to be raised and soon."

The fan mail that came in was extraordinary—it literally came by the bagful and contained every proposition known to man. These ran all the way from the man in Manitoba who had a sure-proof way of making millions which he was willing to give to me at no charge, if I would just get him a lawyer to get him out of jail on a murder rap, to the young lady in Quebec City who wanted a patron to assist her to continue her studies and who sent along a nude photo to assist me in making my decision. There were eight proposals of marriage and about thirty related propositions, while many of the letters came from infuriated insurance salesmen and irate stockbrokers who wished to point out the error of my ways. But most writers were just plain anxious to make a buck and their letters could be summarized by "What's good in the market?"

The book was an incredible financial success. It ultimately sold 187,000 hard-cover copies — 150,000 more through the Book of the Month Club and two million soft-cover through Bantam Books. Six years later it was still selling a respectable one thousand paperbacks a week and in 1973 I issued a revised edition which brought the advice up to date. Unfortunately this attracted the attention of the U.S. Securities Exchange Commission who now wrote me requesting that I register as an investment adviser.

I was flattered at the U.S. government's belated attention and replied that if they thought I was an investment adviser I would be happy to oblige them. Their response was to send me a twenty-five page form to fill out. Question one asked what were my qualifications to be an investment adviser and because I hated to put down "none," I asked my lawyer's advice. He warned me not to register because with my lack of qualifications the SEC would probably refuse me registration and then as a rejected investment adviser they might move to prevent sale of my books.

After reading the regulations which had come with the SEC material I wrote back to them declining to register, claiming I was exempt under this regulation because (a) I had less than fifteen clients, (the only person I gave advice to was my wife and she didn't follow it anyway) and (b) I didn't hold myself out generally as an investment adviser.

This reply upset the SEC and they thundered back: "Compliance with the federal securities act is no laughing matter." They then proceeded to point out the various horrendous penalties they could exact from me—huge fines and long jail sentences for each copy of the book I had sold.

And that's how it ended (up to now at least) because the only way they can get compliance with their orders in Canada is to send in the marines. I suggested to the premier of Ontario that he show support for a fellow citizen by using his fleet of fire-fighting planes to carry out a pre-emptive water bombing strike on the SEC building in Washington, but he didn't think that would make them change their minds.

Governments don't seem too different anywhere.

Anyone Can Make a Million carried on its jacket the words, "How one man parlayed $400 into a million," but in the book itself I didn't relate the actual story of how I made my money and instead wrote individual chapters on the various forms of investing with advice on each.

My own beginning in the stock market was remarkably unsuccessful. It's true that I began with $400 but I managed to lose $350 of that in my first trade. In 1949 I was engaged to be married and my fiancée confided in me that her wealthy cousin, a famous Toronto stock promoter, had given the family a tip on his latest wonder, a penny dreadful by the name of Duvay Mines then trading at 17 cents and "certain to go to a dollar by Christmas." I was young, impressionable and stupid and I could hardly wait to "invest" my $400 in Duvay. By Christmas Duvay was down to 2 cents and as my new father-in-law put it to me, "He should have called it Oy Vay." I sold out, recovered $50 of my investment and dimly began to perceive that there was more to investing than bad tips.

My second venture was far more successful. By the spring of 1950 I had painfully built my bank account back up to $300, and was anxious to try again. One day there was a front-page story in the *Toronto Star* relating a huge new copper discovery down in the Maritimes and the article concluded "Mr. J. Boylen, discoverer of the new mine, has named his company Brunswick Mining and is issuing stock to the public at $16 per share. Brokers on the street indicate that it may begin trading at much higher figures." I phoned Mr. Boylen and told him that I would like to buy one hundred shares of his stock. He said that would be fine and did I want to send a cheque or would I prefer that he deliver the stock to my broker against payment. I quickly suggested that the latter idea would be fine (not having the $1600, I had very little choice).

I now phoned Cliff Lowe, my next-door neighbour and a stockbroker with Doherty Roadhouse and Company, and explained my problem to him. Cliff laughed and said "not to worry—that stock is already $20 bid. I will sell it for you immediately and we will send you the $400 profit after we get delivery."

I had never dreamt that money could be made so easily and I quickly phoned Boylen back intending to order another hundred shares. No such luck, for he was allowing only one hundred shares to each applicant, so I became very busy phoning all my friends and relatives asking each of them to order one hundred shares of Brunswick Mining from Mr. Boylen and promising each one $100 for his phone call. Before the day was out I had made $8000, had a stake to work with and had picked up a million dollars' worth of knowledge in the form of the secret of "free riding," or the purchase and sale of stock without the use of money.

My next venture was in the field of government bonds. At that time interest rates were falling, which meant that new bond issues rose in price before payment date arrived. Using my $8000, I purchased eight new government bonds and resold them the next day at a small profit. No one asked for payment for the bonds and so I began trading larger and larger amounts. Within three months I was doing blocks of bonds as large as a quarter of a million dollars at a time, and within a year I had made close to a quarter of a million dollars in this way. I never looked back.

Strangely enough, I made my largest profits in areas where I was not trying to make money at all. By 1954 I had made a lot of money and the excitement of stocks, bonds and commodities had begun to fade and I decided to buy some "name" art to grace my home. Today I remember with embarrassment the day I walked into Blair Laing's Toronto gallery and asked to purchase "some impressionist paintings." Mr. Laing brought out a Rouault, a Utrillo and a Dufy and after a cursory glance I said, "Okay, wrap them up, I'll take them." The dubious gallery owner insisted on delivering them. I am sure he wanted to see if my cheque would bounce before he parted with his paintings.

I followed this casual purchase with that of a small Renoir and some years later sold three of these paintings and used the profits to buy a lovely home in downtown Toronto.

Money per se has never been terribly important to me and I have made and casually spent vast amounts. What is important is the freedom it has given me to be my own man and go my own way.

The other delegation I received that February day was equally off-beat. CBC producer Ron Weyman and writer Philip Hirsch told me that they had been intrigued by the newspaper publicity I had been receiving and would like to produce a fictionalized documentary series for CBC television about my exploits. Would I help them by opening my files to give them story ideas? My excitement and enthusiasm overcame my business sense and I quickly said yes without even bothering to ask for a royalty.

Stratford veteran actor John Vernon landed the plum role as the coroner. "Morton Shulman" was changed to "Steve Wojeck" and a pilot program was made about an unscrupulous contractor whose deliberate disregard for safety regulations in a tunnel excavation caused the death of immigrant Italian workers.

Now, fearing the worst, I gingerly approached the Attorney General's office to tell them of the new project and seek their approval, but they seemed quite indifferent and so we steamed ahead. The pilot was largely shot in the morgue (unfortunately in order to save money, the CBC used 16mm black and white instead of colour: this penny-wise attitude ultimately cost them dearly because it prevented resale to the U.S. networks) and it went very well. When it was screened for the media there was universal praise; in fact, the only sour note came from me—I didn't approve of the commercial sponsored by Chrysler in which they boasted of the speed of their latest model car. But my criticism was far outweighed by the praise from everyone else. In fact the Toronto *Star* reviewer, Roy Shields, said the first Wojeck play was "probably the best television play ever produced in Canada."

The series now proceeded to programs on the drug problem, on jailing of teenagers with hardened criminals, on suicide in a jail cell, on abortion and on the "sacrifice" of a policeman after he was "crucified by a stupid newspaper columnist." The one subject the program avoided was automobile deaths resulting from faulty construction until finally at the end of their first series I needled the CBC publicly, asking if they were afraid of their sponsors. This got action and they filmed a pretty tough program on that very subject.

"Wojeck" quickly went to the top of the Sunday night ratings and its great success resulted in a follow-up series the following year and a sale of both series to the Australian government network and the BBC. After the BBC had run the twenty programs they decided to run a twenty-first on the real Wojeck and sent a crew from England to make a film in and around my home and office. This resulted in an avalanche of fan mail from England, including dozens of letters from Englishmen asking me to investigate various social ills in the British Isles!

"Wojeck" left everyone better off; the writer and producer made a great deal of money, John Vernon became famous and graduated to Hollywood, and I was left with a flock of happy memories. My one disappointment was that I never appeared in the series. I've always wanted to be an actor and I asked if I could have a walk-on part — or at least play a body. I received a half promise but never did get my chance to act.

The Attorney General's department was less enthusiastic about "Wojeck"—the series continually showed the officials as blundering dunderheads and they were understandably annoyed. As one of them put it to me, "We may be stupid occasionally, but we're never *that* stupid."

16 *To Mongolia*

I have always been intrigued by the east, both far and near. Since my childhood it has represented to me everything that was mysterious and exotic and in the late fifties I indulged this passion with a series of trips to Japan and China, to the Soviet Union and down through Tashkent to Afghanistan, Pakistan, India and Nepal. Three goals remained beyond my reach — Outer Mongolia, Birobidjan and Tibet.

In 1965 I persuaded my wife Gloria to accompany me on another Asian jaunt. I wrote the Mongolian ambassador in London, England and, much to my amazement, received prompt approval for a thirty-day visit to Mongolia the following summer. Mongolia lies between Siberia and Manchuria and the only practical method of entry is through Moscow and Irkutsk. Looking at the map I saw that I was going to be tantalizingly close to the legendary Birobidjan.

Back in the nineteen twenties when anti-semitism was beginning to rage in central Europe, Palestine was largely closed to immigration and the Russian communists, in a bid to win the sympathy of world Jewry, set up a "national homeland" for the Jew in the Soviet far east. Birobidjan was then a frozen wasteland lying on the Arctic circle, inhabited only by a few Eskimos and accessible only by the once-a-week Trans-Siberian railway whose trains did not even stop as they steamed through. Lenin declared that this area was to be given to the "Jews of the World" and the

Soviets invited Jews everywhere to come to Birobidjan to settle and to have their own province and their own homeland.

One hundred thousand Jews came from the starving Ukraine, an area then still tormented by "White" raids and pogroms, and a few thousand others came from other parts of the Soviet Union. Another few hundred came from outside Russia, idealistic pioneers who despaired of receiving justice and equality anywhere else.

At first Birobidjan flourished, a synagogue was built, a Jewish daily newspaper was established and the largest library in the world of the books of Jewish humourist Sholem Aleichem was built. Periodically, sympathetic western Jews visited Birobidjan and sent back glowing reports of a bustling Jewish city surrounded by a province of Jewish farmers.

All this ended abruptly in 1937 with Stalin's purges and the new wave of Soviet anti-semitism. Suddenly the propaganda out of Birobidjan ceased. Visitors were no longer welcome and a curtain came down on the province which has never been lifted.

I determined to try to visit Birobidjan since I was going to be so close. I began my efforts in the usual way with an application to the Soviet embassy in Ottawa. This produced an immediate "Nyet," so I contacted my local MP, Stan Haidasz, and asked him to intervene through our Minister of External Affairs, Paul Martin. Mr. Martin wired the Canadian ambassador in Moscow and asked him to make a request to the Soviet foreign ministry. This produced a more polite "Nyet."

In 1957, when travelling in Russia, I had met one Vladimir Smirnoff, a most unusual Russian diplomat who had later arrived at my home in Toronto in 1963 bearing gifts and followed by an entourage of RCMP secret service men. Smirnoff said his function was to encourage friendship and travel between the Canadian people and his countrymen but, unlike other Russians, he travelled alone and had large amounts of money. I was convinced he was a spy, but I didn't care as I had no secrets to hide. He spent several evenings with us that summer and then returned to Moscow to a post in the foreign ministry.

I now wrote to him reminding him of his visit and asked him to do me a favour and arrange a visa for Birobidjan. He wrote back that he would like to help but there was "unfortunately no hotel in Birobidjan" and so the city was closed to tourists.

I made my last effort through reporter Ted Steubing of the Toronto *Telegram*. Dimitri Polyanski, the Soviet Vice-Premier was then touring Canada and Steubing had been assigned the job of travelling with him on behalf of the *Telegram*. One night Steubing approached Polyanski's aide, told him that an important Canadian official wished to visit a Russian city and was having difficulty. The aid replied, "No problem—give me the details and I'll arrange it." Steubing gave him the information and the next day a crestfallen aide returned to say that he was very sorry but it was just not possible.

I had now exhausted every possibility and I reluctantly abandoned all hope of visiting Birobidjan. We were due to leave Toronto for Moscow on July 2 and the night before had gone to bed early but were woken at midnight by a long distance call. The strange caller identified himself as George Popov and said he was phoning from the Soviet embassy in Ottawa. He was happy to inform me that our Birobidjan visas had been granted but since there was no time to have these entered in our passports we would be given them during our Moscow stopover. Mr. Popov did not say who had arranged the visas.

When we arrived in Moscow we went straight to the Canadian Embassy but they were astonished at our arrival and told us that the visa had been rejected. We then went off to the Ministry of the Interior and they said that they had no information on the matter but would inquire and that when we reached Ulan Bator we should visit the Soviet embassy.

The visit to Mongolia turned out to be a nightmare. Mongolia is a huge land the size of western Europe with only a million people scattered over its flat steppe. When we arrived the capital, Ulan Bator, was suffering the effects of a flood which had knocked out the rudimentary electrical and water supplies. Most Mongolians live in tents called yurts and were barely affected, but the modern six-storey Czech-built hotel was in chaos—the dining room was crippled and the stench from the bathrooms appalling.

Before leaving by jeep for the Gobi desert and South Gobi, we visited the Russian embassy, where I hopefully asked the ambassador if our visas had arrived for Birobidjan. He said that he had heard nothing but he would wire Moscow for instructions and on our return from the Gobi we should come back to the embassy.

For the next ten days we travelled across Southern Mongolia by jeep. We saw thousands of animals tame and wild — horses, camels, goats and sheep — visited innumerable yurts and drank gallons of kumis, which is fermented mare's milk. But because of the flood there were no fruit or vegetables available and on our strange new diet of mutton three times a day I began to sicken. After ten days I had developed all the signs of scurvy, with general weakness, loosening teeth and bleeding gums. Finally I could go no further and took to bed in a yurt, fully convinced that I was dying. I told Gloria not to attempt to ship my body home but to bury me in the Gobi.

At this low point salvation arrived in the form of our driver who had somewhere procured a can of vitamin-enriched pears and fortified by this delicacy I struggled from my bed. There was no way I could jeep back to Ulan Bator and the Mongolians sent what appeared to be a pre-World War I biplane to pick us up. The flight was memorable. The plane had no seat belts, or seats for that matter, and eight passengers sat on benches facing each other with a huge vomiting pot placed between us. All six Mongolians used it liberally.

Back in Ulan Bator I tottered off to the Soviet embassy but, no, they had received no word from Moscow. The ambassador was a friendly man and he was sympathetic to my obvious upset. Why did we want to go to Birobidjan, anyway? "There is nothing there anymore." When I explained that it was a life-long dream, he unexpectedly said, "Well, I think that you are wasting your time —but if you really want to go I'll give you a visa," and as simply as that he took our passports and wrote in the magic words!"

The next day we flew to Irkutsk, the capital of Siberia, and there transferred to a plane for Khabarovsk. This city sits on the Chinese border at the terminus of the Trans-Siberian railway (Vladivostok is a little further but was then a closed garrison city). We arrived in Khabarovsk at 9:00 P.M. to discover that no one spoke English and no one expected us. And so we sat in the airport for two hours until finally an interpreter arrived. We told her that we were bound for Birobidjan and would like to board the next train in that direction. To our amazement the interpreter replied, "unfortunately all the other tourists have already left for Birobidjan. I will take you to a hotel and tomorrow we will see."

The next morning we rose early and hurried to the tourist office. There the official in charge glared at our passports and informed us, "Birobidjan is closed — no one goes there — I must wire Moscow for instructions. Meanwhile go and see Khabarovsk." That morning we went sightseeing and at lunch the tourist official informed us, "I am very sorry but you cannot go to Birobidjan — there is a convention there and the hotel is full."

Now I finally lost my temper and I roared at him, "I have not come all around the world to get within a hundred miles of my goal and be turned away. I am going to the railway station now and I am boarding the first train for Birobidjan and if you wish to stop me you must arrest me," and then I threw in the clincher, "And if you do I shall order my government to stop all wheat shipments to Russia."

Amazingly, this hollow threat worked. Within one hour we were supplied with an English interpreter and were on our way to the railway station. The interpreter, a Jewish girl called Fagel, was as excited as we were. "I have lived my whole life here and have never been to Birobidjan."

After all our struggles Birobidjan itself was anticlimactic. It is a decaying provincial Yiddish town. The population of 100,000 is now only half Jewish, although all the signs are in both Russian and Yiddish (Hebrew is not allowed). The town produces agricultural machinery and shoes and has a huge agricultural market and a technical university. But there is no regular university and the young people are encouraged to move elsewhere. There is a daily Yiddish paper and the editor proudly displayed his collection of foreign papers to prove that he received a cross-section of information from around the world. They consisted entirely of Communist papers like New York's *Daily Worker* and Toronto's *Tribune*.

A broad range of books published in Yiddish were sold, contrary to what I had been told in Canada, and the Yiddish library contained over 100,000 books. We asked the newspaper editor to take us to the synagogue and he at first refused saying that no one went there. Finally, when we insisted, he took us to a dilapidated tiny building at the edge of town—the rabbi had died and not been replaced but there was a cantor and we left a Jewish prayer shawl with him.

There was, of course, no convention in Birobidjan—in fact we were the only visitors at the hotel, which was very primitive. This was the real reason visitors are discouraged from visiting Birobidjan; Russia likes to show off her best, not her worst. Birobidjan is an experiment that failed.

17 *Shulman v. the U.S. Navy*

Every year one of the most popular crowd pleasers at the Canadian National Exhibition is the air show in which air stunts, the latest planes, formation flying, trick flying and air deviltry are shown off for the benefit of thousands of watchers. For several years the bravest and most daring part of the show was put on by the Blue Angels, the acrobatic team of the air arm of the United States Navy, who swept in close formation across the waterfront, wings almost touching, the planes going at the speed of sound.

On September 2, 1966, in the middle of the show, one of the Blue Angel planes, piloted by Lt. Commander Richard Oliver, crashed near the huge CNE audience, scattering its wreckage along five thousand feet of the airport runway. Commander Oliver died instantly but fortunately no one else was injured. The events that followed the crash were chaotic.

The airport lies on a small island in Toronto Bay and the audience were seated on bleachers on the waterfront looking out towards the lake. Immediately after the crash took place, reporters and photographers started to cross to the island by small boat or on the ferry. There they were halted by a colonel of the United States Air Force who ordered them off the airfield. "We've had a plane go down and this is now American territory," he announced. The colonel was backed up by several other US officers and a contingent of Toronto police. The sergeant in charge of the police detail said he was taking his orders from the US officials on the scene: "And if you don't like it, I'll get off this motorcycle and make you like it," the police sergeant roared.

Just then a Canadian air force officer arrived and requested that the journalists be allowed to visit the crash site but the US officers flatly refused him and they ordered the police to "clear them out."

Meanwhile I had received a call from the morgue telling me that there had been a plane crash and death at the island. So I went down to the waterfront, commandeered a boat from the harbour police and arrived at the island just as all the reporters were being herded off. I examined the shattered remains of Commander Oliver and ordered his body taken to the morgue for an autopsy. By now it was getting dark and I didn't feel anything more could be done at the scene, so I ordered the police to take charge of the wreckage and said that I would return in the morning.

The next morning I attended the autopsy at the morgue and then returned to the island airport. The wreckage had all mysteriously disappeared from the runway and I was told that some twenty-three police officers had walked abreast for twelve hours along the five-thousand foot runway collecting every piece of metal and that it had all been put in a corner of the huge hangar. I went to the hangar where I was astonished to find a team of seven orange-coated American technicians sorting out the wreckage. The leader introduced himself as Commander Harry Walker and I immediately asked him, "Why are you working at this instead of the RCAF?" The commander replied that his team consisted of experts and specialists who would be far more familiar with this type of plane. This appeared reasonable to me and I replied, "Okay, you go ahead—when will I get your report as to the cause of the crash?" Commander Walker then said, "That is not possible. Let's sit down over a cup of coffee."

We went to the lunch counter where Commander Walker told me that he was responsible only to the US navy and could not possibly let me know what he found from his investigation. I then explained to him the function of the coroner and that I must know the cause of the crash in order to be able to make reasonable suggestions to prevent a recurrence. The commander said he was sorry but he could not give me the information. I then told him that if he would not cooperate he would have to remove his men from the hangar.

Both of our tempers were now rising and Commander Walker informed me that he had no intention of leaving until his investigation was completed. My reply to this was to call over the Toronto police sergeant who was in command of the twenty-three man detail. "I am taking charge of this wreckage under the authority of the Coroner's Act—escort Commander Walker and his men out of the hangar and if they attempt to touch the wreckage again place them under arrest for interfering with my warrant."

The seven US navy men, red-faced with anger, changed from their bright orange fatigue suits, put on their uniforms and silently filed from the hangar. As he walked out, Commander Walker said to me, "You will be hearing from Washington about this."

Now I had possession of the wreckage but did not have the faintest idea what to do with it. As a first step I made out a subpoena for Commander Walker to attend the forthcoming inquest and ordered the police to serve it upon him at once. They rushed to the Skyline Hotel where he had been staying, but there learned that Washington had ordered the team to return to the United States and they had already left for the airport. The police officers hurried over to the airport but arrived just after the Americans' plane had departed.

My troubles quickly mounted. Commander W.J. Gable of the US Navy said that the Navy's encounter with me "had been a shock" and that "people usually have more respect for the navy of the United States of America." A spokesman from the Canadian Ministry of Defence in Ottawa said that Canada and the US had an agreement that investigators probe their own crashes on foreign soil. The *Telegram* chimed in, "Dr. Shulman's behaviour is really atrocious. Any incident sufficiently serious to ruffle the feathers of Canadian officials and American experts should be referred to Ottawa where the facilities for dealing with such things are available and adequate. Dr. Shulman must recognize the difference between a mishap to an American tourist on one of our highways and a tragedy touching a branch of the armed services of our closest ally."

Meanwhile the heat was mounting on me, as the press kept calling to ask who was going to investigate the wreckage. I phoned the RCAF to ask for their help and the next day three beribboned air force officers arrived in my office to give me the bad news. They said that:

(1) They were not familiar with the aircraft involved, a Grumman Tiger, and had no one who could intelligently examine the wreckage.

(2) Ottawa had advised them that the investigation should be done by the US authorities.

(3) If I would apologize to the US team, the Americans would return and complete their investigation but they could not create a precedent by giving me, or an inquest jury, the results of their findings.

I asked the air force men if there was anything about the plane that was a military secret and they replied, "No—nothing at all," and I then said to them: "Okay, you go back to Ottawa and tell your boss that unless you people come up with experts to examine this wreckage or alternatively the Americans come back to do it themselves and give me their report, I am going to the Russian consulate and ask them if they have experts who can help me. I will give you 48 hours."

Two days later the Canadian Ministry of Defence issued this statement. "Group Captain Edward Boland, Commanding Officer of Canadian Forces Base, Toronto, was asked by Dr. Shulman to provide some technical assistance so a report can be given at the inquest into Lt. Commander Oliver's death. On Monday morning Group Captain Boland led a three-man medical and flight safety team to the island and made an investigation."

I was quite amazed at the furore that had blown up. Newspapers both in Canada and the United States were full of letters praising my independence (Canada) or condemning my "disgraceful actions" (USA). One comment that tickled me was written by Scott Young in the *Globe and Mail*: "I would like to have had a transcription of the thoughts of the United States air crash investigation when they met Metro's Chief Coroner. There is no doubt that on occasion Dr. Shulman acts with a sense of authority otherwise found only in beings which come out of a bottle in a puff of smoke, but we can stand a few of these around (I guess)". The letters from the United States were all very much alike. My favourite was written by one Victor Griffin and appeared in the *Toronto Star*: "It is obvious Dr. Shulman saw a chance to further his political career by a cheap sleazy appeal to those Canadians who get their patriotic kicks by twisting the US lion's tail. Coroner Shulman and those Canadians who gleefully applauded his despicable action in stopping this investigation have stooped to a new low. Inherent in any public office is a requirement for dignity, civility and sane conduct. Dr. Shulman's actions ignore these. Thank God I'm an American."

At the inquest, Alan Frye, the Department of Transport Director of Operations for the CNE show testified that at the Blue Angels' rehearsal the day before the crash, the Americans' wing tips were only ten feet above the water while the RCAF always kept to a minimum two hundred feet. Mr. Frye said that he had alerted the Angels' team commander about the low flying but he said the warning may never have reached the pilots. Frye also admitted that the dead pilot had had "several drinks" at a late-night party the evening before the crash—Oliver had left the party about 2:00 A.M.

Despite numerous requests, no representative of the Blue Angels or the US Navy appeared at the inquest, but the Canadian experts testified that there was no indication of any mechanical fault in the airplane.

The evidence revealed that there had been five CNE airshow-connected deaths since 1949 and that it was just a lucky fluke that hundreds of people had not been killed in the crash. The jury deliberated for some hours and then recommended that in future a minimum height of two hundred feet be allowed for air shows. Within a week the CNE announced that it had accepted the jury's recommendation and had instituted a two-hundred-foot minimum. There has not been a CNE air show crash since that date.

There was an unusual postscript to this story. After the RCAF team had completed their investigation of the wreckage a single police officer was left there on guard on each shift. After several days of this boredom the officer on day duty was offered a ride in a small Cessna by one of the private plane owners. The policeman injudiciously accepted the offer and the owner crashed on landing. The plane was a complete wreck, but miraculously neither man was injured and the new mass of wreckage was left piled up beside the smashed US Navy Grumman. After the inquest the US authorities asked if they could have their wreckage back and a few days later a van arrived to take it away. Unfortunately in the confusion they shovelled up the metal from both planes and shipped it off to Washington.

I've often wondered what their report said after the US experts had sifted through that shipment!

18 *Outside My Jurisdiction*

Unbeknownst to me reporter Gerald McAuliffe of the *Hamilton Spectator* had been visiting inquests in Hamilton (which was completely out of my jurisdiction). His observations had included one inquest where the coroner fell asleep during the proceedings, another where the jury consisted of five court constables, a third where the court constable wrote the jury's verdict because the coroner was in a hurry to get away, and three subsequent inquests conducted by the same coroner in which they completed the evidence in the first inquest, started the second inquest while the jury was out, then adjourned it when the first jury was ready to come back, resumed the second inquest, and then started the third inquest while the jury was out.

McAuliffe was pretty upset by all these shenanigans and he phoned me in Toronto asking me to send him a copy of the Coroner's Act and any other rules that we had regarding conduct of coroners. I mailed the material to him and dismissed it from my mind. After receiving my package McAuliffe went to Hamilton's St. Joseph's Hospital to question a senior doctor he knew there about the coroners in Hamilton. The doctor was very unhappy about the entire situation and casually mentioned that a few weeks earlier a woman being treated for severe burns had died from an overdose of blood transfusions in his hospital and that the matter had been covered up. McAuliffe was very excited by this story and searched his paper's record for a list of women who had died in the previous three months in St. Joseph's — there were thirty-five names. He now went to the Vital Statistics office but was refused permission to examine the death certificates.

At this point McAuliffe called me again, gave me the list of names and asked if I would be willing to find which woman had died from the overdose. I agreed and called him back the next day to report that it was one Edith Somordolea and the death certificate had been signed by Hamilton Coroner Dr. Bulford. (The certificate did not mention blood transfusions but did mention the burns and congestion of the chest.)

McAuliffe now called Dr. Bulford and told him that it was his understanding that Mrs. Somordolea had been admitted to hospital with severe burns in August and had died three weeks later after receiving an excessively large blood transfusion. Bulford hung up on McAuliffe after the latter suggested that the death certificate had been incorrectly filled out. McAuliffe then telephoned Dr. Connell, the Chief Coroner of Hamilton, but he did no better there, for Dr. Connell merely said that in his opinion he didn't believe it was a matter that warranted an inquest.

The next day, January 18, 1965, McAuliffe phoned Supervising Coroner H. Beatty Cotnam and told him the story; Dr. Cotnam said he did not believe an inquest was necessary and, furthermore, he went on to say that he did not believe that an investigation should be launched each time a reporter called him. Following the conversation McAuliffe phoned Attorney General Arthur Wishart and told him everything that he had told Doctors Bulford, Connell and Cotnam, and also that Dr. Cotnam did not believe the matter warranted further investigation, but that he, McAuliffe, was convinced that the death certificate was false and that an investigation was warranted. The Attorney General replied that he would order an investigation and instructed his deputy to find out what was going on.

Meanwhile the *Hamilton Spectator* published a series of articles about the death of Mrs. Somordolea and quoted Dr. Cotnam as saying that the lady had died of natural causes and no inquest was necessary.

Four days later, in a letter to the Assistant Deputy Attorney General, Dr. Cotnam wrote that after receiving the medical records "it is apparent to me that there is sufficient grounds for an inquest which should have been held in the first place." He requested a direction to conduct the inquest himself.

Gerald McAuliffe had singlehandedly forced this inquest on the basis of fairly skimpy information. What he did not know was that the Death Review Committee of St. Joseph's Hospital had met after Mrs. Somordolea's death with both Coroners Bulford and Connell in attendance. The final lines of the minutes taken at this meeting read as follows: "Dr. Bulford, the coroner assigned to the case, stated he felt this patient probably might well have died from other causes. The Medical Director pointed out that it was the coroner who phoned him and stated, 'This patient should be alive today.' The decision reached by this meeting was that the death was not preventable. The Chief Coroner stated that neither he nor Dr. Bulford had mentioned a word of the case to anyone outside of Hamilton and he urged that no details of this case be conveyed to the press."

Following this meeting the hospital's Medical Advisory Committee met and ordered that the hospital privileges of Mrs. Somordolea's physician be restricted.

If I had used reasonable prudence I would have stayed strictly out of this whole mess, but instead I foolishly jumped into the fray. On January 18, I called Dr. Bulford (who answered two or three questions and then told me to mind my own business). I then wrote the Attorney General suggesting that something was very wrong and concluded: "This case appears especially serious because Dr. Bulford assured me today that Dr. Cotnam was aware of all the facts and that a copy of Dr. Bulford's report had been forwarded to Dr. Cotnam." I had received no reply to this letter when it was announced that an inquest would be held and would be conducted by Dr. Cotnam. I exploded in another letter to the Attorney General, "If Dr. Cotnam presides at this inquest there will be a grave suspicion that this case is being whitewashed. I hope you will make other arrangements."

At the inquest six specialists gave evidence. Dr. Eydt, a specialist in internal medicine stated that he personally would not give a patient this quantity of blood. Dr. Yaworski, the hospital pathologist, gave his opinion, "that death was precipitated by a blood transfusion." Dr. Goldberg, the head of the department of medicine, gave his opinion that the blood contributed to her death. Dr. Lane, the head of the department of surgery, said that he would not have given "this amount of blood over the time period in question." Dr. Osbaldeston, the hospital Chief of Staff, said that "this death was preventable, and there was an error in judgment." Finally Dr. R.A. Haygar, the head hospital pathologist, stated, "Blood transfusion was precipitating factor in death of patient."

After hearing all the evidence Dr. Cotnam told the jury: "The coroners involved in this case decided that no inquest was necessary and after hearing all their evidence I agree with the original decision—it would appear to boil down to a difference of opinion in treatment only."

He said that the Attorney General had directed an inquest "not necessarily because he disagreed with the coroners' decision regarding the inquest, but rather because of the many nasty and vicious complaints and rumours involving the doctor and also the coroner in this case, and the Attorney General decided that an inquest was necessary to clear the air and he directed me to hold this inquest for that purpose . . . "

The jury attached no blame to anyone.

My interference on a matter entirely outside of my jurisdiction had infuriated the Attorney General and this was soon to cause me considerable trouble.

In the meantime another suspicious death was brought to my attention. On November 27, 1964, sixty-six-year-old Mrs. Pearl Gray had died in Toronto's St. Michael's Hospital from a generalized infection which had begun following surgery for haemorrhoids in a small town near Barrie. Her death was investigated by Coroner Elie Cass and by the local police and on December 11, 1964, Dr. Cass sent me a copy of the police report with this cryptic note attached, "After reading this over you may form the conclusion that some form of skullduggery was involved in her treatment."

The facts were indeed disturbing. The physician involved was a general practitioner who had attempted to remove Mrs. Gray's haemorrhoids but had been unsuccessful and perforated her rectum (the pathologist's report said the rectum had been perforated but that *no* surgery had been performed).

The physician had a prior history of alcoholism and drug addiction and had recently been returned his hospital privileges after a six-month suspension.

I forwarded all the facts I had available to Dr. Cotnam and recommended that an inquest be held and he assigned Dr. Shannon, a local coroner, to carry this out. On January 7, 1964, I wrote Dr. Shannon and suggested that he look into all of these matters. After making investigations Dr. Shannon was satisfied that the doctor had not been under the influence of alcohol or drugs at the time of the operation. As to the doctor's previous problems, Dr. Shannon did not bring them up at the inquest because he found that the man had been previously suspended by the College of Physicians and Surgeons for a period of six months and his licence had been then restored, and "when the College restores someone's licence they are very sure things have been corrected."

On January 20, 1965, the inquest was held and the jury brought in this verdict: "Death was caused by peritonitis . . . We do not find that any negligence has been proven. We recommend that the press should refrain from passing an opinion." Dr. Cotnam had sat through the inquest and was sufficiently surprised by this that he remarked to the press, "I don't see how the jury arrived at its recommendation—possibly small town sensitivity had something to do with it." The mystery was solved very quickly. The jury foreman, R.J. Franks, a local trucker, commented that he felt the whole affair had been "a trial by newspaper" for *his* doctor. It took only a few minutes for me to discover that each of the five jurors had used that particular doctor either as his own physician or for the medical care of his family. As one of the jurors put it, "I was not biased. I wanted to be certain of the integrity of my physician and if he did not have integrity I wanted to know about it and therefore I went into the inquest with my eyes open."

Dr. Cotnam had not been aware of the composition of the jury until after the inquest and although he said it was "a little out of the ordinary" he did not feel being a patient would disqualify a man from jury duty as there was nothing in the Coroner's Act against it.

On January 21, 1965, I made the serious blunder of writing to Attorney General Wishart asking that a new inquest be held because the jurymen were all patients of the doctor concerned and because the presiding coroner had not raised the matters I had brought to his attention. The Attorney General replied the next month and gave it to me with both barrels:

> There are certain fundamental principles of our society that are fundamental not only to the administration of justice but also to the civil rights and liberties of all the citizens of this Province. It is fundamental that any person who is accused of misconduct either of a civil or of a criminal nature must be brought before a court of competent jurisdiction in order that he might not only have full knowledge of the charge but also that he may be given the opportunity to defend the charge, or cross-examine witnesses, to call witnesses, and to submit argument to the court. In the course of any such proceedings the rules of evidence are adhered to to ensure that there are no unjustifiable excursions into areas that are not relevant to the charge. In your letter of January 7th to Dr. Frank Shannon of Barrie, you took it upon yourself to suggest that certain questions be asked and that certain determinations be made which, in my opinion, had no relevance whatsoever to the purpose of the inquest. The questions were not only irrelevant in that context but they were of a nature that would not have been admitted in any court of law. Questions relating to the past conduct of the attending physician with additional questions suggesting misconduct on a prior occasion because of alcoholism or drug addiction could completely ruin the reputation of the physician in this forum where he has no legal rights whatsoever to defend himself against these innuendos and their possible implications. This is even more unreasonable when I am advised that the evidence at the inquest affirmatively established that the attending doctor appeared to be completely normal at the time of the operation and there was absolutely no suggestion that he was impaired in

> any way. I am not aware of any circumstances which would justify the type of question you suggested to Dr. Shannon, and if there is any justification, would you let me have it.

I should have shut up but I fired a letter right back to him:

> The questions which I requested to be asked at the inquest were to establish that if the medical authorities . . . had done their duty and notified the College of Physicians and Surgeons, disciplinary action would have been taken and this operation would not have taken place and the patient would be alive today. This could be most important in preventing further operative deaths. The most important point was of course that this was a biased, improper jury, headed by a foreman currently a patient of the doctor involved.

I received no reply to this last effort.

19 *The Poison Epidemic and Other Symptoms of Notoriety*

Beginning in early 1965 and rising to its peak in mid 1966, the Coroner's Office had a rush of over one hundred individuals who came to us complaining that they were being poisoned. These people were of all ages and from every walk of life. Although none of them knew of the others they all had remarkably similar stories. Invariably they had gradually developed symptoms of illness over a period of weeks and simultaneously noticed a bitter taste to their food. They all had come to the same conclusion, which was that they were being poisoned by relatives, friends or neighbours. At first I took their stories at face value and for some months we kept the crime lab busy analysing things like pork pie and birthday cake, but it finally dawned on me that we were finding no poisons and besides no one was actually dying. What Toronto was undergoing was an epidemic of "poison delusions" — the sort of thing that had taken place fairly commonly in the Middle Ages.

On a few occasions I suggested that the "victims" see a psychiatrist but this produced a very hostile response — these people were completely rational on every other subject and flatly rejected any suggestion that their problem was anything but physical. I tried tasting the foods myself in front of them but they were not convinced. "You'd get sick if you ate it every day."

We finally found a solution to our problem — we referred them to the police, the police sent them to the municipal Department of Health, the Health Department referred them to the Crime Lab, the Crime Lab referred them to an independent lab, the independent lab sent them to the provincial Department of Health, the department suggested they see their family doctor, he sent them to us and we sent them back to the police.

It sounds foolish but it actually worked. The persons suffering from these delusions were quite happy to make the rounds and present their bags of poisoned dover sole or ham and eggs to the various officials they met. The running about from office to office burnt up their excess energy and gradually these delusions faded. By late 1966 the poison epidemic had almost disappeared.

Incidentally 105 of the 110 "victims" were women.

In fact, I seemed to attract the attention of an amazing quantity of mentally sick people. I couldn't believe the number of strange letters, both tragic and comic, that poured into the Coroner's Office every day. Some people were convinced that their loved ones had been done in by foul play or they themselves were threatened.

> I am well satisfied that the two doctors conspired together on the night or some time on February 26th to kill my husband with a stab in the jugular vein in the throat and two other stab wounds on the right side of his neck from 'needle rejections' inflicted some time after our daughter and I had paid a visit to the hospital.

> May I ask you to send me a letter of reference. Every man has a right to earn a living and Canada is a land of the free. Dr. – – is a lunatic. He inflicts cruelty on people. He is cruel to me.

> Suppose that my niece was done to death by the forces of organized crime because she possessed inside knowledge from babyhood up but had ceased to be (from their point of view) a 'reliable' person; suppose that I am not a neurotic old woman but a person who is being attacked by the same forces because I steadfastly refuse to go along with what has happened and is happening. My sister-in-law may be in similar danger though for a different reason. Whilst she has tried to do everything demanded of her she had a lifelong genius of making bad mistakes . . . I quote verbatim from her letter re her 'fibrola-

tion'. I had another attack of this fibrolation which went on and on and on while I was at make-up course (in connection with amateur theatricals). Most embarrassing. But they were so good to me.

I fear we Canadians are headed for a sorry state of affairs in this our centennial year and in the years ahead.

On September 21st, 1962 the late G– N– ... stated that for the last twenty years practically all of the deaths in Ontario have been caused by call girl leaders such as the late Reverend Johnston, the late Harold Rowe, old Betty, and the Brewins witching up a flood of dope stealers to force drug addicts to murder friends and relatives with germ warfare, heart attack pills without antidotes, depression, dope, fast driving, dope, goof balls, etc.

Others were anxious to bring about improvements for the world at large.

Since the biologists tell us that trout young are full of life and move about before there is any cardiac action it is reasonable to suppose that the reverse is possible and that even after the legal 'mortality code' conditions are established there is still some life left and the sensation of pain may exist for a long time ... I am hoping to get legislation enacted so that an autopsy can only legally be performed with the written consent of the most important party in the proceedings i.e. the corpse.

My aim is to make cremation sound as attractive as possible. One look at the coroner's building on Lombard Street and the rude, seedy-looking bunch of men inside hardly inspires confidence. One can only feel dismay that this important seat of justice is degrading to everyone concerned ... For some people the 48 hour delay for cremation presents a worry. To be blunt —odour from a dead body begins on the second day. Under our present system only embalming will make the presence of bodies bearable until the third day. I understand that in many European countries the problem is relieved by refrigeration. Would it be possible for refrigerators to come into use here and for undertakers to be fined for embalming against the wishes of the family.

> Are you acquainted with the benefits of deep breathing? . . . I began practising deep breathing in 1958 and since that time have never lost my tremendous enthusiasm for it . . . I'm convinced if people would try it for one month every day they would note a marked improvement in their conditions . . . I should be out working every day . . . however I cannot bring myself to it, this conviction that deep breathing has such tremendous potential and could help so many fills me with an unrelenting desire to instruct in its attainment.

> I need your assistance, sir. Airlines must carry parachutes. I have given the advice to CPA . . . the Titanic taught a lesson at sea . . .

Some were suffering from strange or rare diseases.

> Have you heard of a person contracting a disease from domestic rabbits? . . . Every doctor has said nerves, your age and the aftermath of a hysterectomy. It may sound like that but with a whole herd of rabbits affected every ninety days at the same time I get sick, make me wonder what it is. For one thing is certain none of them ever had a hysterectomy and they have no worries to cause nerves. . .The reason I am writing is that I have had rabbits affected with this die after being fed medicine or even malt lavall and if I really do have what they have, I hope no one says allergy, cancer or what-have-you, if my heart stops undergoing these tests. Every rabbit I have opened up has a flabby heart, damaged lungs and hemorrhaging. Bowels are so swollen they are obstructed. They show no signs of pain nor do I . . . Rabbits are listless as end nears and usually go out with a slight convulsion. Maybe I am worrying unduly.

The deputy chief psychiatrist at the Queen Street Ontario Hospital advised me in 1967, that there were 40,000 psychotic persons at large in Toronto alone. "Most of them are harmless," he reassured me. It was his theory that the unusually high proportion of mental illness in southern Ontario is a result of the excessive inbreeding that took place among the United Empire Loyalists.

Another side effect of all the publicity I had been receiving was that I was approached repeatedly by various hucksters seeking to use my name to sell one thing or another. One of these gentlemen, a Mr. Sol Allen, was very persistent. Allen had made a small fortune in the picture theatre business and had used this money to indulge his vanity as a writer. He had written two books about doctors but because no publisher would accept them he had set up his own publishing house and cranked them out. The books were badly written sexy horror stories about doctors' incompetence and they had barely any sales. Allen was determined to try again.

On April 15, 1964, Sol Allen phoned me and told me that he had just completed an exciting new book, *The Gynecologist*, that he wished me to read; if I would agree to it being published as having been written by the two of us he would give me the first $50,000 of royalties. I went to his home that evening and picked up the manuscript and went home to read the first fifty pages. The book was indescribably badly written and within a few minutes I knew that I wanted nothing to do with it. I should have just phoned him and said no, but I foolishly wrote Allen a letter politely turning him down.

On July 11, 1965, I was approached by Allen's lawyer, a Mr. Gerald Soloway, who told me that Allen wished to use the letter which I had sent to him to advertise his book and would pay me $500 for this privilege. I replied that under no circumstances would I agree to this and Soloway then told me that he was afraid that Mr. Allen was going to use it whether or not I gave permission. I said to Mr. Soloway that I thought this was very immoral and he agreed.

On July 17, 1965, the *Globe and Mail* carried a full-page ad for Sol Allen's new book, headlined "The book the establishment tried to suppress," and underneath this a reproduction of my letter reading "Very reluctantly I have come to the conclusion that even with massive changes I could not associate myself with it. I am truly sorry."

I'm not sure which made me more angry—the implication that I had suppressed this terrible novel, or being called "establishment." In any case I roared off to hire a lawyer and by some strange happenstance chose one Charles Dubin, boy genius, director of the *Telegram*, and darling of the Tory party. Dubin advised me that a lawsuit would just give Allen the publicity he was seeking and advised me to drop the matter.

I reluctantly agreed and no one ever heard of Allen again but my contact with Charlie Dubin was not over by a long shot.

20 *Suicides and Drugs*

Suicide was the one form of death I could never come to terms with. Natural deaths, accidental deaths, homicides — these were all something with which one could do battle, but the taking of one's own life has always been that great inexplicable. Life to me is so precious that I cannot conceive of anyone voluntarily surrendering it and each suicide I had to investigate deeply disturbed me.

Prior to 1963 it had been the practice in Ontario to conceal suicides "for the family's sake" and so the rule had been laid down that unless an actual suicide note was found, accident or natural causes was put on the death certificate. I reversed this ruling and from 1963 on, accurate statistics were kept. This resulted in an immediate apparent dramatic jump in the number of suicides which was understandable; but what was not so understandable was that the number of suicides continued to grow each year after that until by 1965 there were 175 suicides in Toronto — a larger figure than the number of traffic deaths. The following year a new policy was introduced of holding inquests in every case in which there appeared to be a possibility of preventing similar deaths through public exposure and recommendations. We had immediate positive results. In 1965 a series of deaths had occurred after attempted suicides were given first aid in hospital emergency wards and were then sent home where they repeated their suicide attempts more successfully. These repeated attempts quickly declined after publicity from several inquests resulted in the Toronto hospitals referring attempted suicides to psychiatrists.

I was fascinated by the variety of methods used by suicidal persons and the cross-section of society that was afflicted and began to study the suicide notes, hoping to find a pattern. There was none. Some were pathetic scrawls, others carefully worded statements. Marital discord, loneliness, paranoia, suicide pacts—the motives were as various as the people themselves.

Beginning in 1965 we ran into a series of drug-induced suicides and toward the end of 1966 several cases occurred of young men killing themselves by jumping from high places after taking LSD. LSD was then an entirely new drug which no one knew much about. There were no laws governing its possession or use and the papers were full of incredibly euphoric tales by individuals who had tried it. Among the youth subculture it was believed that this was the ultimate "trip", while at the same time these stories were balanced by hysterical "Ban LSD before it's too late" speeches from the politicians.

On January 4, 1967, the body of a twenty-eight-year-old poet, Henry "The Man" Borycki, was found on the Don Valley golf course beneath the Hoggs Hollow bridge. At the inquest which followed a series of witnesses gave evidence that Borycki was a very unhappy youth who regularly took LSD because this removed his depression "and made him serene." Sunny Gale, Borycki's best friend, swore that Borycki had sought psychiatric help for his depressions at several Toronto hospitals but that they had all turned him away.

Mrs. Kay Johnston, Borycki's former teacher, said he was "the soul of honour, the finest young man I ever taught and thousands have passed through my hands." Eric LeBourdais, a freelance writer, testified that he had been researching material for an article on suicides to see what help was available for would-be suicides. "One Sunday night I made twenty-three calls to different hospitals and agencies. I cited the fictitious case of an aunt of mine who I said was deeply depressed and in need of professional help. All my calls were fruitless. I had replies ranging from 'We have no psychiatrist on duty,' through 'call this number please and try there,' to 'If she becomes violent bring her in and we'll give her a shot'."

The jury recommended that a Metro crisis centre be set up where emotionally disturbed persons could receive help.

The Borycki inquest was barely completed when another LSD death took place. Twenty-year-old John Stern, a talented young composer, had been fascinated by the writings and speeches of Timothy Leary, the high priest of the LSD cult. On March 18, 1967, Stern had obtained a quantity of LSD and, together with a seventeen-year-old friend, rented a hotel room and swallowed the drug at 3:00 P.M. The younger boy said he did not take the drug because Stern had asked him to be a witness while he took it experimentally: "John went on a trip and saw flashing lights—he was really high." Later in the day the boy said that Stern went into a deep depression and around 8:00 P.M. they went home. They took a taxi to the younger boy's home and he went indoors, leaving Stern outside. One hour later John Stern plunged to his death from the Bloor Street bridge onto the Don Valley Parkway. I ordered that an inquest be convened for April 11 and instructed the police to attempt to determine the source of the LSD.

Young Stern's father was understandably bitter. He told the press, "There's not the slightest doubt that disciples of LSD contributed to his death, his murder. So does every publication that in any way glorifies this drug as a magic gift that can broaden and enlighten anyone. The fact is that LSD holds a lure for the brilliant and gifted of our young. They listen to the glowing and glittering tales of its ability to reveal to them a world of brilliance and vision. They are not told of its dangers. That's why I hope that every physician, every authority, every publication and everyone with an influence on young people will take Johnny's death as a symbol to demand the utter and total prohibition of LSD except by qualified medical research people."

Meanwhile I felt that in order to intelligently advise the jury I should know what this drug was all about and so decided to try it myself. I contacted a friend with connections in Yorkville and she brought me a little tablet about the size of a pin head. The next Sunday at 4:00 P.M. I swallowed this tasteless odourless little pill and wrote the following note and placed it in the bureau in front of me:

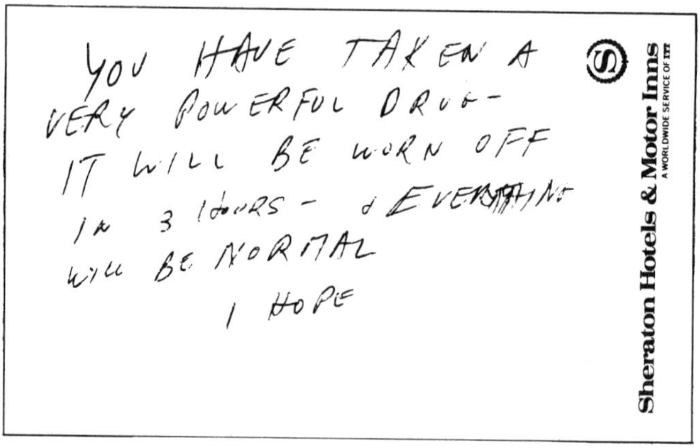

YOU HAVE TAKEN A
VERY POWERFUL DRUG-
IT WILL BE WORN OFF
IN 3 HOURS - & EVERYTHING
WILL BE NORMAL
I HOPE

Sheraton Hotels & Motor Inns
A WORLDWIDE SERVICE OF ITT

By 6:00 P.M. nothing had happened and I was convinced that the whole thing was a fake. At 7:00 P.M. I started seeing flashing lights and re-wrote my note,

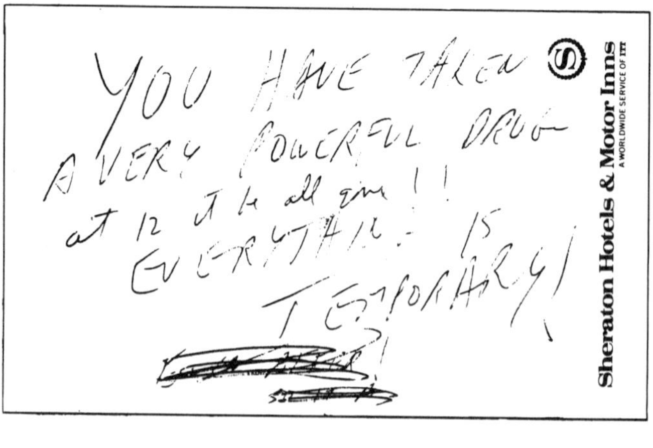

YOU HAVE TAKEN
A VERY POWERFUL DRUG
at 12 it be all over!!
EVERYTHING IS
TEMPORARY!

Sheraton Hotels & Motor Inns
A WORLDWIDE SERVICE OF ITT

By 8:00 P.M. I was quite out of my mind—I had lost the senses of touch and rational sight and could barely write.

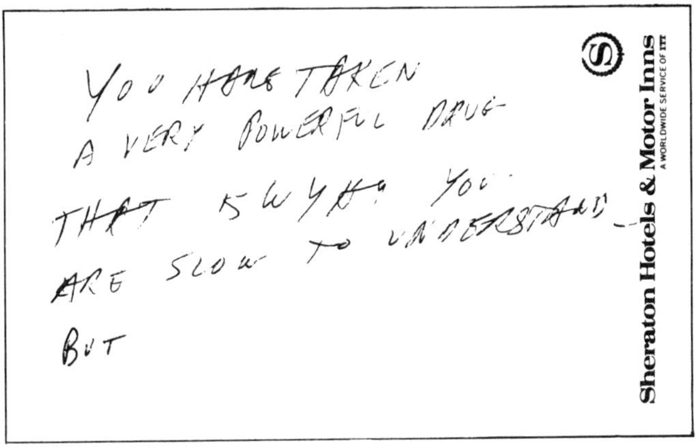
YOU HAVE TAKEN
A VERY POWERFUL DRUG
THAT IS WHY YOU
ARE SLOW TO UNDERSTAND
BUT

Sheraton Hotels & Motor Inns
A WORLDWIDE SERVICE OF ITT

I thought that I was one of the characters in a television movie playing in front of me and attempted to attack one of the other characters on the screen. I had to be restrained and then assisted to my bed.

By 11:00 P.M. it was all over. I determined to advise the Stern jury to recommend that LSD be banned.

The events leading up to the inquest were hardly reassuring. On April 7 the police brought me a list of the witnesses to be called at the inquest with a summary of their evidence. The following note was attached to the police statement: "As to the source of supply to the deceased of LSD, this matter is still under investigation and it would not be deemed advisable to divulge the results of the investigation to date in this vein for obvious reasons."

The reasons were anything but obvious to me so I phoned the home of the officer in charge of the investigation, and asked him why there was no evidence available as to the source of the LSD. The police sergeant replied that the inquest should not look into that aspect of the matter at all but should confine itself to investigating what Stern died of and the circumstances preceding his death. I disagreed but could not persuade the sergeant to change his mind so then went on to ask him why the youth who had been seen with Stern at the time he was believed to be buying the LSD had not been subpoenaed. He replied, "We have been unable to locate him. We think he has gone to Montreal."

It just didn't ring right, so I phoned police headquarters and asked the duty officer to dig out the index of inquest witnesses and to give me the phone number of the young man in question and he promptly did so. I then phoned the number and to my amazement the young man himself answered the phone. I said to him, "I would like very much to speak to you about the death of John Stern. May I come up to your house?" He replied, "Yes, if you wish."

By now I was quite disturbed so I phoned the sergeant back and asked him, "Do you think that this youth could be a lead to the source of the LSD?" and he replied, "Yes, but unfortunately he is in Montreal. We have no way of getting to him."

I then phoned Sergeant Roy Norman, the police officer assigned to the Coroner's Office, and instructed him to prepare a subpoena for the young man. Then the two of us went together to his home where we served it upon him.

Later the mystery deepened when I was phoned by one David O'Brien who had actually witnessed John Stern fall from the bridge and had given a statement to the police but had been told not to appear at the inquest. I instructed him to attend.

The next problem was to find an expert on LSD who could give impartial evidence at the inquest and I didn't know where to begin. Finally I phoned Princeton University because they had done a great deal of research on this drug in the previous two years. There I spoke to the head of the department, Dr. Humphrey Osman, and I asked him to come to Toronto to give expert evidence. He replied, "Why call me when you have the leading man in the world in your own country, Dr. Abraham Hoffer?" Following this advice I phoned Dr. Hoffer at the University of Saskatchewan and he agreed to come to Toronto to attend the inquest.

All of this was done for nothing—the day before the inquest was to convene I was served with an order-in-council dismissing me from my job as Chief Coroner and the provincial government moved immediately to take over the Stern inquest. Abraham Hoffer was told not to come to the inquest and the subpoenas I had served were cancelled. When the inquest convened Fred Cruikshank, the elderly assistant coroner who sat on the bench, read a statement to the jury. "The issue in this case is not where the material was obtained or whether it was obtained illegally. These matters are for investigation by the police." Later Dr. Cruikshank admitted that he could not recall ever before giving such instructions to a jury and also admitted that he had done so as the result of a conversation he had had with an official in the Attorney General's department.

No one ever did determine the source of the LSD.

21 *Third Time Unlucky*

The end of my career as a coroner came suddenly following a fire at the "fireproof" Downsview hospital of the Workmen's Compensation Board. On March 20, 1967, fire had broken out in that hospital and before it was extinguished a patient, Francesco Gualtieri, had burned to death. Dr. Elie Cass was assigned by my office to investigate the case.

The following morning I was phoned by Don Delaplante, a veteran *Globe* reporter, who told me that he had just visited the Workmen's Compensation Board Hospital where he had discovered that the supposedly fireproof hospital had been built with an inflammable cardboard ceiling, that the plans had not been submitted to the Fire Marshall's office before building commenced, that the building had not been properly inspected during the eight years it was up and that the patients had been taking night leave and going to a nearby bar and getting back in the hospital by climbing through windows. He went on to warn me that since this was a government-built hospital and the Minister of Labour, Dalton Bales, had given speeches about its modern fireproof construction, this case could affect the expected upcoming election and that I should keep a close eye on it. I had been then dealing with Delaplante for over ten years and I knew him to be both conscientious and reliable and so I immediately phoned Dr. Cass to alert him. He informed me that he had ordered an inquest to be held on May 2.

On Monday, April 3, Jack Hills, Dr. Cotnam's assistant, phoned Dr. Cass and told him that Dr. Cotnam was taking over the case and intended to convene a jury for April 4 to visit the scene of the fire. Dr. Cass immediately reported this to me and I blew up.

Back on February 28, 1964, at the time of my first public battle with Arthur Wishart the matter had been smoothed over after my interview with the Premier, when Elliott Pepper, the former Queen's Proctor, had been called in as a go-between. He had met with Bill Common, the Deputy Attorney General and had then sent Mr. Common a letter, a copy of which he gave to me, which said in part: "I have also explained to [Dr. Shulman] that it is mutually acceptable to everyone that in the future both Dr. Shulman and the supervising coroner will follow proper channels in all matters so that if the supervising coroner is concerned about any matter arising in the County of York he will contact Dr. Shulman rather than individual assistant coroners and Dr. Shulman will follow the same procedure."

From that time until the Workmen's Compensation Board fire I had certainly stuck to this agreement and so far as I knew so had Dr. Cotnam — certainly he had made no effort to take over any inquest and to my knowledge had never on any case gone around me to any of the individual assistant coroners.

This intervention now coming on the heels of Don Delaplante's phone call made me suspect the worst and I jumped to the conclusion that the government was sufficiently embarrassed by the fire that they intended to try to cover up the facts and prevent a full investigation.

Looking back I feel that I was wrong and that Dr. Cotnam had no such instructions or motive. I suspect that things were very quiet at the Supervising Coroner's office that week and he was merely looking for an interesting case to work on. But veteran Queen's Park reporter Harold Greer had a different theory. "From all the available evidence here, it seems clear that Dr. Cotnam was finally determined to assert his jurisdiction over Dr. Shulman and was simply forcing the issue knowing that Dr. Shulman would probably react (one does not have to observe Dr. Shulman for long to predict his behaviour) in such a fashion that the government would have no alternative but to fire him."

In any case, I instructed Dr. Cass that he was working under my direction and I ordered him not to relinquish the inquest but to convene it as soon as possible and I would send him a letter giving him the appropriate authority. I followed this up by ordering the police officers in our employ at the Coroner's Office that the facilities of the morgue were not to be made available to Dr. Cotnam for the purpose of holding such an inquest.

I now made my final fatal error by sending this letter to Attorney General Wishart.

> You will recall that in April of 1965, at the time of our most unfortunate public fracas, an agreement was made to prevent any future recurrence. At that time I undertook to make no public comments respecting cases occurring outside of Metropolitan Toronto, that I would release no critical comment of this department or its officials and that I would communicate with the department through the Supervising Coroner. Up until this moment I have taken care to comply with my portion of the agreement although there have been certain occasions particularly involving cases in other jurisdictions which in my opinion required comment. In return I requested that Dr. Cotnam not interfere in the work of the Metro Coroner's Office nor call individual Metro coroners re their cases.
>
> Last week a fire occurred at the Workmen's Compensation Hospital, in which preliminary inquiries indicate that there may have been negligence on the part of provincial authorities. One of our more able coroners, Dr. E. Cass, was assigned to investigate the fire and to hold an inquest. This has been set for April 5th, 1967. Today Dr. Cass was called by Mr. Jack Hills instructing him not to hold the inquest and saying that Dr. Cotnam would hold one in his place. Inasmuch as this is in direct contradiction to our agreement and in addition carries the unpleasant implication that the government does not wish all the facts brought out, I have issued instruction to Dr. Cass to continue with the inquest and have so instructed the police; barring a direct order from you to the contrary.
>
> If I receive such an order I shall understand that our agreement of April 1965 is no longer in effect.

As soon as he received the letter Arthur Wishart determined to fire me and he marched into the Tory cabinet meeting that morning with an ultimatum for the unhappy Premier Robarts. "There is only one course to follow, gentlemen. I don't think we can live with the man anymore. I don't think we can put up with him any longer. Either Shulman goes or I quit myself. If that man stays in that job, the government might just as well crawl into a hole and hide its head." There was a mild attempt to dissuade the Attorney General but he was adamant and the cabinet gave him the okay reluctantly, very worried about the effect on the coming election. Arthur Wishart had one minor problem in that the estimates for his department were then before the House and if my firing were made public he knew that the opposition parties would make it a major issue. He therefore held up the announcement while the debate on the estimates ground on, but was put on the spot by the Liberal justice critic Vernon Singer, who asked him what was going on. With a straight face Mr. Wishart replied, "The Chief Coroner for Metro Toronto is being informed that the Supervising Coroner of Ontario has supervision and control over all coroners and that he must respect the advice and supervision given by the Supervising Coroner for Ontario." Outside the House the Attorney General announced that he had in his briefcase a letter to be sent to me containing a rebuke for my actions. He later said, "Shulman has many qualities I admire, but loyalty isn't one of them."

Meanwhile Dr. Cotnam gave a statement to the press. "This death was not being properly investigated until I intervened and under no circumstances was I undertaking a whitewash. I have never whitewashed anything since I was appointed the Supervising Coroner 5 years ago. . . . Every year for 5 years Dr. Shulman has broken out into the same kind of tirade. It's a broken record that keeps repeating. He likes to bathe his ego in publicity. He has again demonstrated his ability to distort facts. Dr. Shulman is a man who likes to look like a knight in shining armour and thinks of himself as the only person who can dispense justice."

On April 7 Attorney General Wishart's estimates were through the legislature and on that day he sent his letter off to me and simultaneously informed the press that he was doing so. That afternoon I was attending a Coroners' Conference at the Westbury Hotel. Thirty coroners sat in a cramped little room discussing methods of more accurately determining the exact time of death in a corpse, when a knock came at the door. One of the coroners came over to me and told me I was wanted.

I said, "Well, tell them I'm busy."

He replied, "They say it's urgent."

I went to the door and found an official government messenger who handed me a sealed letter marked personal, confidential and urgent. Standing in the hall I opened it and read my dismissal.

> Dear Dr. Shulman:
> I received your letter of April 3, 1967. Your defiance of the Supervising Coroner for this Province is not only completely unwarranted but a repudiation of The Coroner's Act and my office. Your innuendo that this Government does not wish to have the facts brought out impugns not only the integrity of my officials, but also the Government and constitutes an attitude that is quite inconsistent with the responsible and judicial character of the office of Chief Coroner.
>
> Your appointment as Chief Coroner for Metropolitan Toronto and as a Coroner for the County of York has therefore been terminated as of this date.
>
> In view of the statements which you have made respecting the inquest into the death of Francesco Gualtieri, I have given instructions that you are to be subpoenaed before the inquest in order that you may disclose any facts or information that you deem relevant to the inquiry.

There seemed no point in returning to the coroners' meeting as, on this case at least, the time of death seemed clearly established.

When I got back to my office I began to study Mr. Wishart's letter. If the common law books were really correct and "the coroner is an independent functionary responsible only to the public," then surely I could not be fired just by the Attorney General writing a letter. I had been appointed by an order-in-council signed by the Lieutenant-Governor and so I insisted that I could only be fired the same way. Meanwhile I kept possession of my office at the morgue and announced that I intended to conduct the Stern LSD inquest which I had already set for April 12. On April 11 I was presented with an order-in-council dismissing me.

I should not have been surprised that I was fired, but I had been misled by Arthur Wishart's mild statements in the House, and so presumed that once again everything would blow over. To say that I was in shock at losing my job would be a great understatement and in my first flush of anger I proceeded to make the biggest mistake of my whole life.

Looking back with the benefit of hindsight I now realize that I should have accepted my dismissal gracefully, said I was sorry but I'd done my best and quietly retired. This would have saved me untold aggravation, harassment and expense. Instead of this I fired back at the government with everything I had and opened my files to the press, thus revealing all my charges of previous coverups and mismanagement dating right back to the Pisecny inquest. The publicity that followed was horrendous and the media headlined all of my charges of coverup, of whitewash, of waste and of ethnic discrimination. Premier Robarts was appalled and on Monday April 10 he announced that a royal commission would be appointed to investigate my charges. It was essential to the Tory government that my charges be disproved and that I be discredited as quickly as possible. Perhaps it was coincidental that the intended spring election was postponed to the fall.

On April 11 a fracas developed in the legislature after Arthur Wishart rose on a question of privilege to attack Jim Renwick, the NDP justice critic who had charged the Attorney General with slyness for bringing in an amendment to the Coroner's Act the previous year which gave the Cabinet the power to fire coroners by an order-in-council. Before that amendment was passed, Mr. Renwick had said, coroners could only be fired on evidence of misconduct. Mr. Wishart labelled Mr. Renwick's accusation base and snide. "To suggest or infer that this was a deceptive or deceitful ploy by a responsible minister is a gross and complete distortion of both law and fact." In the uproar that followed, angry NDP members demanded the right to reply to the Attorney General's charges and when NDP member Ken Bryden refused to sit down, the seventy-five-year-old Sergeant-at-Arms B. Handly Geary rose from his seat on the floor of the legislature and approached Bryden's desk, sword clanking and medals bristling. "Sit down," shouted Mr. Bryden at the white-haired Victoria Cross winner, "Are we to be subjected to the rule of force?" Geary backed up a step, called Bryden "an insolent pup," and returned to his seat. All the members were screaming and it was with great difficulty that the Speaker restored order. Later, when poised beside each other in the washroom, the Speaker remarked to Donald MacDonald, the leader of the NDP, "It's amazing how there could be so much fuss over one pushy Jew."

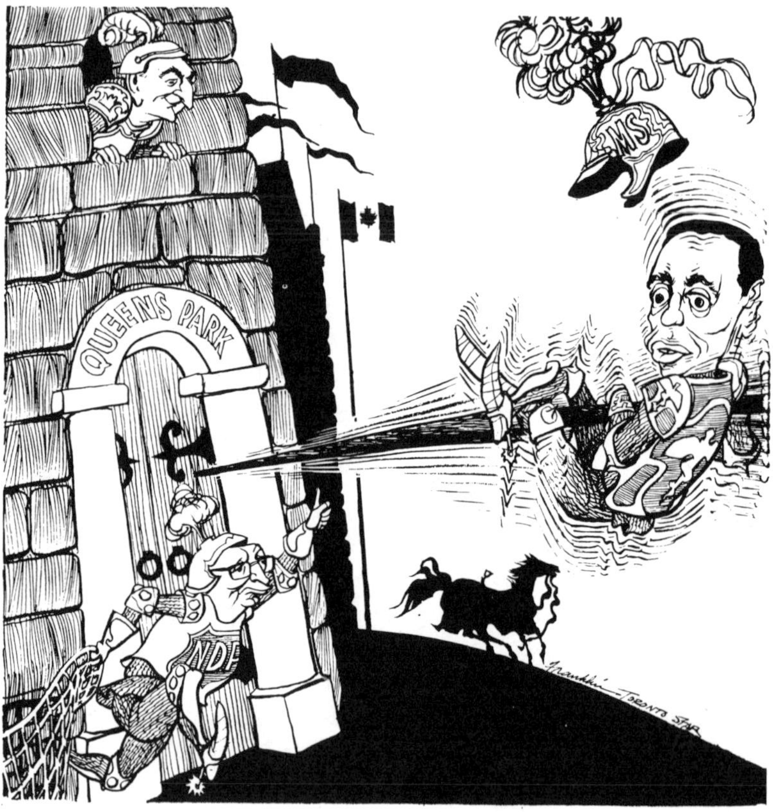

22 *The Royal Commission*

The aftermath of my firing was quite extraordinary. The Labourer's Union placed a picket line in front of Queen's Park in protest, thousands of letters and telegrams poured into my office and also into the offices of Premier Robarts and Arthur Wishart, and in the legislature there were screams of protest from both opposition parties who demanded (but were refused) an emergency debate. My phone was constantly busy with hundreds phoning in to volunteer their help if I decided to run for office and both opposition parties sent emissaries to offer their support and to seek my allegiance.

I had been overjoyed when Premier Robarts announced that there was to be a royal commission to investigate my charges. In my naïveté I prepared a 125-page brief containing all the details and assumed that I would be allowed to present this brief, would be then cross-examined by government lawyers and that the obvious truth would result in my vindication. I could not have been more wrong. Actually I received my first hints almost at once with warnings from my more politically aware friends. Also, as early as April 14, Ron Haggart wrote in his column in the *Star*: "Now we are to have a judicial inquiry, an inquest into the coroner's own demise. And we shall wait, just like the patient good gray men of government, and we shall see whether it is to be a bold and penetrating inquest, or whether it is to be an inquest of the kind we used to have."

The very next day I learned the bad news. Chosen as commissioner of the inquiry was Mr. Justice William D. Parker of the Supreme Court of Ontario and former president of the Hamilton West Progressive Conservative Association. I expressed my dismay immediately. "I would have hoped the Premier might have picked a jurist who had not held such a prominent position in his party." Judge Parker responded, "If Dr. Shulman is implying this will affect my judgment I have no comment to make. I don't relish the work but I think it's my duty to take it."

Chosen as commission counsel was none other than Charles Dubin. I went back through the *Globe and Mail's* clipping file and found that he had acted as special counsel for the Attorney General during the hearings on the Ontario highways scandal in which construction companies had defrauded the public of some millions of dollars and following which Farquhar Oliver, then leader of the Liberal party said that for his services, "Mr. Dubin should get a title from Queen's Park for the work he did for the provincial government." During the Northern Ontario Natural Gas scandal Dubin had been a defence lawyer and at that time was quoted as saying. "It is no offence for a person in office to receive a gift." Somewhat more reassuring was a speech he had given just one year earlier to the Law Society in which he spoke of the deep inequities of royal commissions.

As the registrar of the commission the Tories picked H.W. Biggar, former president of the Toronto Central Progressive Conservative Association.

My growing pessimism about the commission hearing deepened. When I met with Mr. Dubin and he asked me to detail my allegations, I agreed provided that he would present them or allow me to present them in order and in total. He flatly refused and our conversation concluded on that note.

I then made another in my series of errors. A *Telegram* reporter asked if he could have a copy of my brief to assist the newspaper in following the evidence and I gave it to him. That copy was somehow passed on to Mr. Dubin and it lay on the counsel table in front of him as the hearings opened.

Immediately after the hearings began I learned the true nature of the mess I was in—not only was I not allowed to read my brief in order or in total but Mr. Dubin proceeded to put me on the stand on each point and followed each of my appearances with conflicting evidence. I pleaded in vain that he at least take the cases in the order in which they had occurred so that they would develop logically and my actions not appear illogical. When he refused I appealed to Judge Parker, "May I ask that we take the cases in a consecutive way?" The Judge replied, "No."

Worse, I immediately found myself being vigorously cross-examined by Charles Dubin while he treated my adversaries in a more gentle fashion. Here are samples from the first week of hearings:

Dubin: You are suggesting Dr. Cotnam would conduct a mock inquest?
Shulman: Yes, I am.
Dubin: Yes, now he has been the supervising coroner in this province for a long time?
Shulman: Yes, he has.
Dubin: Now in the . . .
Shulman: And let me say he has conducted a lot of good inquests, and I am not suggesting all of them . . .
Dubin: Well that is very judicious of you, after making the strongest slur on a man in public life I think I have ever heard.
Shulman: Sir, may I back it up with facts.
Dubin: You are going to back it up with facts. But I think allegations are not facts. I want to get the facts.
Shulman: Well, let me . . .
Dubin: Just a moment. You will when we get around to it.

Compare that with Mr. Dubin's examination of Deputy Attorney General William Common the following day.

Dubin: Now in your capacity as the Deputy Attorney General of this province did you ever instruct or attempt to unlawfully or improperly suppress investigations or inquests.
Common: Emphatically no.
Dubin: Or interfere with the investigations or and inquests or suppress evidence?

Common: Emphatically no.
Dubin: With respect to any of these matters conducted in the office of the Chief Coroner of Metropolitan Toronto?
Common: Emphatically no.
Dubin: Or any others?
Common: Emphatically no.
Dubin: Well, the suggestion that the Deputy Attorney General of the province would politically interfere and suppress evidence, which was charged against you.
Common: And my officials I might add.
Dubin: And your officials; what do you say about such an allegation as that?
Common: Well, they are completely without foundation . . . I might say, Mr. Dubin and Mr. Commissioner, I resented these implications because there was a strong implication that not only myself but the officials in my department had violated their oath of office with the additional implication of corruption.
Dubin: Thank you, Mr. Common.

I had entered the hearing without a lawyer, believing that the commission had been set up to investigate my allegations and the behaviour of my adversaries and that therefore I did not need a lawyer to help me present the facts. But as the month of May ground on and I was clobbered day after day by Charles Dubin I finally began to realize that I was in effect on trial and that I desperately needed a lawyer if I was to save any portion of my reputation. Just as I began to appreciate my situation Ron Haggart wrote this column in the Toronto *Star*.

> Charles Dubin, who was chosen by Mr. Justice W.D. Parker to present the evidence to him, has said that some of Shulman's language contains the strongest slurs on public men Dubin has ever heard. Shulman has "Impugned the honesty and integrity . . . of everyone associated with the administration of justice," according to Mr. Dubin.
>
> Morton Shulman, by his own choice, does not have a lawyer at the inquiry. Perhaps because of this, he has fared far better in the newspapers than he has at the inquiry; the newspapers are necessarily more concerned with new information and hard

facts than with the mood and the effect of the searching and accusatory cross-examination which Shulman has faced.

The story as it now exists on the record might contain far more material explaining Shulman's actions and his statements to the press if Shulman had a lawyer by his side; the lack of such protection is, however, Shulman's choice.

On Tuesday, Mr. Dubin read into the record quotations from the *Globe and Mail* of Friday, April 7, the most serious being Shulman's statement in the paper that because Dr. Cotnam took control of the hospital inquest "the implications are obvious."

He also referred to another Shulman statement in the same story that inquest plans were already underway before Dr. Cotnam stepped in.

Dubin hammered away with such inquiries as this: "The sinister implication you are making here is that Dr. Cotnam is a man who is not a man of integrity and honesty in the conduct of his office—isn't that what you are saying?"

If Morton Shulman had a lawyer at the inquiry, the lawyer might have pointed out that the *Globe* story containing Shulman's statements which Dubin found so offensive carried an eight-column headline: Shulman accused of lying by Cotnam and reprimanded by Wishart, Mr. Wishart being, of course, the attorney-general and Dr. Cotnam the supervising coroner in his department.

A lawyer might have drawn evidence to show that when Mr. Wishart made his criticisms of Dr. Shulman, Wishart knew that Shulman had already been fired and Dr. Cotnam almost knew.

But Shulman did not know; Shulman was answering criticisms without knowing the true nature of his own position—and all he said was "the implications are obvious" in reply to a man who had called him a liar.

If Morton Shulman had a lawyer at the inquiry he might have read that headline into the record, he might also have read aloud the *Globe's* assessment that Shulman had been subjected to a "stinging attack" from Cotnam the afternoon before. No one else read that into the record.

If Morton Shulman had a lawyer at the inquiry he, no doubt would have pointed out that H. Beatty Cotnam called Morton Shulman a liar and it was in eight-column headlines in the *Globe and Mail*. It was only then that Shulman issued the mild

> rejoinder that the implications of Cotnam's own actions were "obvious."
>
> Shulman's lawyer no doubt would have read into the record the entire *Globe* story with its accusatory headline and strong words about Shulman; and a lawyer would perhaps have pointed out that the rules of decent human behaviour, to say nothing of the laws of libel, allow a man under attack the right of reply.
>
> The entire *Globe* story is an exhibit and Mr. Justice Parker will no doubt read it all and judge the circumstances of Shulman's reply. But if Shulman had a lawyer for himself, he would have put these circumstances clearly on the record.
>
> The fact that H. Beatty Cotnam issued a long press statement on Thursday, April 6, calling Shulman a liar is not even a part of the record of the inquiry, except in the *Globe and Mail* clipping. What is on the record is Charles Dubin's description of Shulman as a man who "slurs" and, "impugns" public officials.
>
> If Morton Shulman had a lawyer at the inquiry he might perhaps soften the impression which so far lies virtually unchallenged — that Shulman was an irresponsible pop-off who called people names in the press. But Dr. Shulman has chosen not to have a lawyer, and he is very much on his own.

Haggart followed this up with a second column in which he examined the curious reasons which were given for Dr. Cotnam taking over the inquest into the Workmen's Compensation Board Hospital fire death, and compared the way the Supervising Coroner's assistant was allowed to tell his story uninterrupted, while I was relentlessly cross-examined. Haggart concluded:

> At every royal commission or judicial inquiry, someone eventually says "No one is on trial here," and it has been said, inevitably, at this one. However much the earnest men in charge of the thing may really believe it, the mood of that muggy room as it appeared to an unlettered layman was that Morton Shulman's reputation was very much on trial, and the prosecution was winning.

I was convinced. I hired Walter Williston to represent me and he promptly appealed to the Court of Appeals to change the procedures whereby Judge Parker and Charles Dubin were running the inquiry. The court ruled in our favour saying that Judge Parker's general procedures in questioning restricted the purpose of the inquiry and were not a "valid exercise of his authority." They also ruled that I was to have the right to examine my own witnesses, but turned down our request that the hearing be confined to charges made while I was Chief Coroner.

Mine was a short-lived victory. The inquiry reconvened July 4 and Mr. Williston could not attend because he was committed to be at an appeal case in Winnipeg. When on July 5 I asked for yet another three-week adjournment so as to find another lawyer Judge Parker refused and said I should have hired a lawyer who was not tied up on other cases. On that note the inquiry resumed on July 10.

23 *How to Become a Socialist*

It was now crystal clear that I would not be vindicated by the royal commission and I determined to take my fight with the government to their own home grounds by becoming a politician. My dilemma was whether to join the Liberals or the New Democrats. The obvious choice was the Liberal party, for my friends were all Liberals, and I believed in free enterprise and had made my fortune in the stock market, whereas my knowledge of socialism came mostly from a murky view of Clement Atlee nationalizing British industry and ruining that country's economy.

My first visit was to meet Bob Nixon, the head of the Liberal party, and he warmly invited me to join his group, offering me the nomination in any of the four Toronto ridings which had not yet chosen a candidate. He concluded that he wanted me to join him even though many of the major Bay Street donors to his party had expressed misgivings. At the very moment that Bob Nixon was wooing me, his front-bench colleague Elmer Sopha was giving a speech in the legislature in which he was putting me in place and was strongly asserting that Arthur Wishart had been right all along. To add to my unease I was approached by a federal Liberal MP who put it on a straight dollars and cents basis and guaranteed me $100,000 as campaign expenses if I would run for his party.

The NDP took a more subtle approach. I was visited at my home by Donald MacDonald, Stephen Lewis and Jim Renwick. There was no talk of money or even of socialism; instead the three men spoke to me of the battles I had been fighting at the Coroner's Office, told me they agreed with all of my stands and said that I would be more effective as part of a team. When I asked which riding I could run in, they told me to take my choice. Lewis said that if I wished he would even give me his own riding of Scarborough West! I could not fail to be impressed by the contrast between these apparent idealists and the realists of the Liberal party—and so by default I joined the NDP. Strangely enough, even though this wedding was arranged without either party really understanding the other it has endured in relative tranquility. On Friday, July 7 I announced my decision at the NDP annual convention. The socialists were overjoyed, the Tories furious, and the Liberals unsure whether to be happy or disappointed.

On July 10 I returned to the Parker Commission and once again asked the judge for an adjournment so that I could find another lawyer. Judge Parker refused saying, "You have been given all the

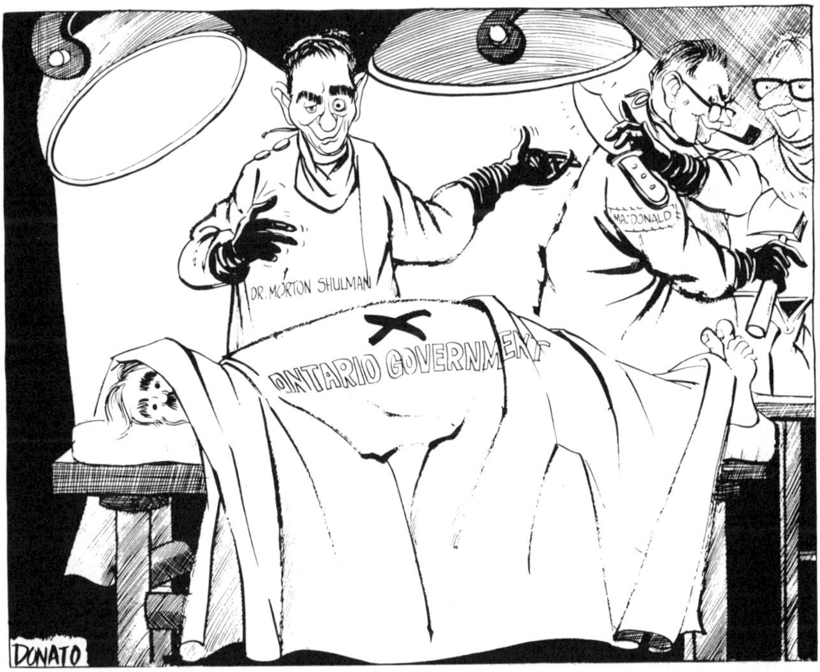

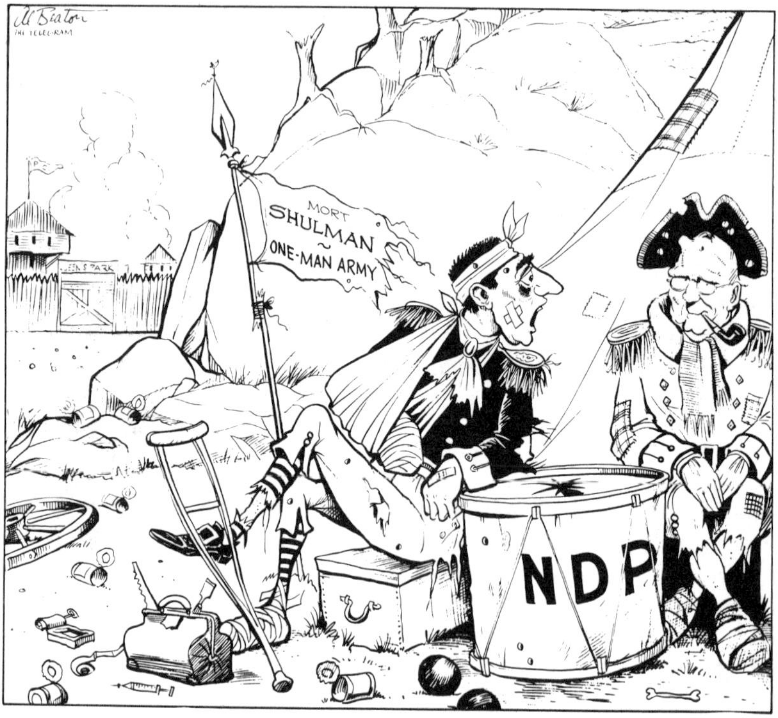

"I'M THINKING OF PLACING MY FIGHTING ABILITIES AT YOUR DISPOSAL."

time in the world but all you want to do is play games. I am getting tired of playing games and I want to get on with this . . . I refuse any more delay, we are going on."

I had tried my best to get counsel but each of the ten lawyers I had approached had said that it would be impossible to prepare such a complex case in the few days available and in desperation I refused to give any more evidence until I was given the opportunity to get a lawyer.

This availed me nothing, for Judge Parker said, "Very well, Dr. Shulman, you realize of course you are here under subpoena and I have the power if I choose to commit you but I do not intend to do so. That would only cause further delay and divert the course of this inquiry."

After the luncheon recess I didn't bother to return but sought out my new allies at the NDP offices for their assistance. I returned

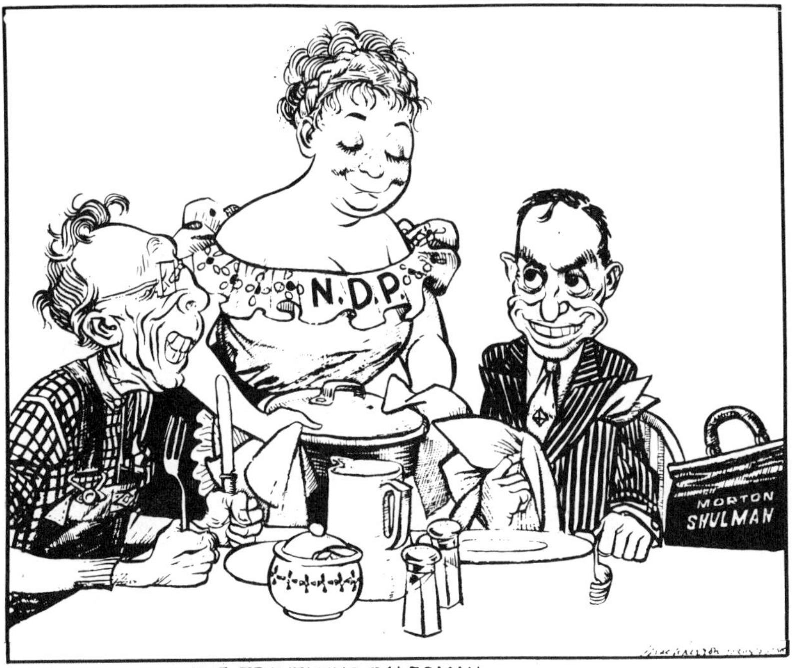
N.D.P.
MORTON SHULMAN

THE TRAVELLING SALESMAN

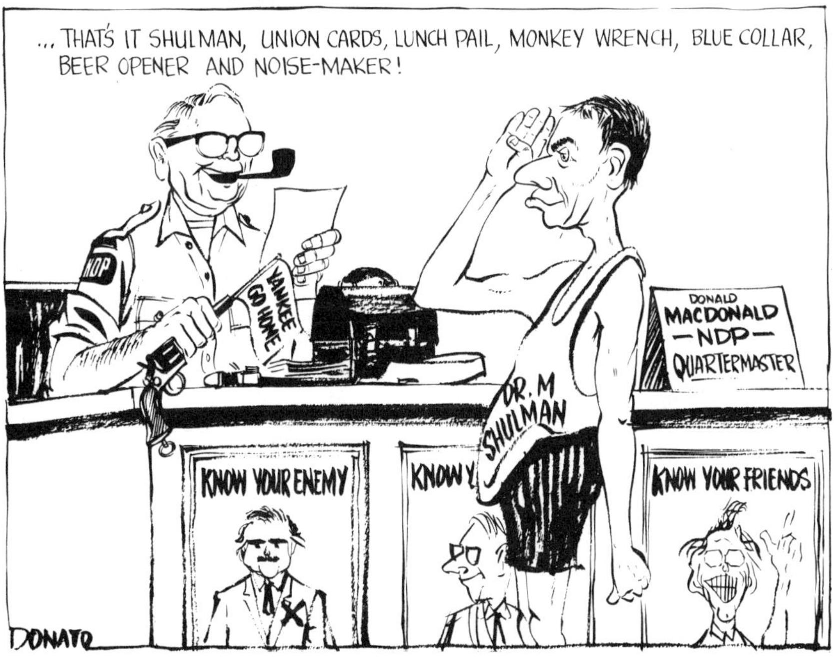
... THAT'S IT SHULMAN, UNION CARDS, LUNCH PAIL, MONKEY WRENCH, BLUE COLLAR, BEER OPENER AND NOISE-MAKER!
NDP
YANKEE GO HOME
DONALD MACDONALD -NDP- QUARTERMASTER
DR. M SHULMAN
KNOW YOUR ENEMY
KNOW Y
KNOW YOUR FRIENDS
DONATO

to the hearing the next morning accompanied by David Lewis, the national leader of the NDP and this resulted in a most extraordinary scene as he pounded the table and dressed down the judge.

> *Mr. Lewis:* Mr. Commissioner, I am here—my name, if you do not recall it, is David Lewis—and I am representing Dr. Shulman. I should add: this morning. I am not at all sure it will be possible for me to continue the case or whether someone else will have to do it.
>
> I am here primarily, may I point out, my lord, because in my respectful opinion from what I have read in the press and from what I have heard from Dr. Shulman and from what I read this morning in the transcript of yesterday's proceedings, a grievous error has been committed; if not an injustice. . . .
>
> It seems to me that it is not unusual for courts and commissions and judges to accommodate clients and counsel. it is not unusual for that to happen.
>
> *The Commissioner:* In fact it is normal provided the client is co-operating and willing to get on.
>
> *Mr. Lewis:* I have read some of this. Let me tell you, Mr. Commissioner, that I am fed to the teeth by this kind of statement from your lordship which I have read. . . .

> *Mr. Lewis:* I say to you it is the duty of this Inquiry to adjourn until—a reasonable adjournment to give Dr. Shulman an opportunity to find counsel.
>
> *The Commissioner:* And do you undertake that if I do grant an adjournment it is not just a stall and you will appear or someone will?
>
> *Mr. Lewis:* I protest in the strongest language. Don't you, Mr. Commissioner, talk to me like that!
>
> *The Commissioner:* I am talking to you like that . . .

> *Mr. Dubin:* I am very much amazed at the intemperate language used by my learned friend Mr. Lewis, for whom I have had the highest regard.
>
> *Mr. Lewis:* And I would be very grateful if Mr. Dubin does not give one of his homilies. I don't need his lectures about behaviour.

The Commissioner: There may be some question about that. However, carry on, Mr. Dubin.

The judge's face had turned scarlet through this exchange and I expected him to jail both David Lewis and me for contempt, but to my utter amazement he meekly backed down and gave Mr. Lewis the very adjournment he had refused me the day before.

It was now perfectly obvious that I was in the position of a well-hooked fish—able to delay the inevitable by vigorous struggling but not able to affect the final outcome. I know now that I should not have bothered with lawyers or appeals to higher courts because these were to cost me dearly in time, aggravation and money and in fact they availed me nothing—the Parker Commission continued regardless on its inexorable way.

I returned to the hearing with E.B. Jolliffe, the former NDP leader, as my new lawyer and the hearing dragged on for several more weeks until finally they ground to a halt with a flurry of charges. Barry Pepper, the lawyer for Dr. Cotnam, called me a wicked man and demanded that I be charged with a breach of the Vital Statistics Act for giving the information on the Somordolea death certificate to reporter Gerry McAuliffe; the lawyer for the Shouldice Clinic urged the judge to probe my trading in the stock market and Brendan O'Brien, lawyer for the Workmen's Compensation Board, called me a bare-faced liar and a public mischief.

Judge Parker did not bring down his report until the following February. In it he ripped me apart saying that I had been wrong on every one of my charges. The terms of the royal commission had been to investigate my allegations of "unlawful or improper suppression of an investigation or inquest," and Judge Parker began his summary as follows.

> The allegations of 'improper suppression of evidence, whitewash and cover-up' are all allegations which imply illegal conduct, since it is a criminal offence willfully to attempt in any manner to obstruct the course of justice.
>
> The submission by counsel for Dr. Shulman that he would not deal with the word "unlawfully" is therefore equivalent to an admission that he could not prove any unlawful conduct. Had Dr. Shulman made this admission at the start of the

hearing considerable time and money would have been saved.

(On the very first day of the hearings Charles Dubin had questioned me as follows:

Dubin: And the cover up you portray is some improper or unlawful act?
Shulman: Not necessarily, certainly not unlawful.
Dubin: You think it is an illegal act.
Shulman: It is not illegal.
Dubin: These are serious allegations you are making.
Shulman: Improper.
Judge Parker: Improper?
Shulman: I think improper is a better word.
Dubin: Not unlawful.
Shulman: Not unlawful.
Dubin: Not illegal.
Shulman: No.)

Judge Parker found that there had not been any improper suppression of evidence in the Pisecny case, in the cancer quack cases, in the Shouldice case, the Somordolea death, the Barbara Moore case or any of the others. He also ruled that there had been no discrimination in the appointment of coroners.

The judge went on to say that I was "glib, irresponsible, unworthy of belief, inconsistent," and finished up his view of my conduct with "smacks of McCarthyism, a technique repugnant."

If Judge Parker's report had been accepted by the public it would have been the end of my political and public life, but strangely enough it had absolutely no effect. Even the Tory government seemed content to let the report be forgotten and it was never quoted in my subsequent political campaigns. *The Globe and Mail* summed it up quite aptly: "The judgment of the public on the battle between Dr. Morton Shulman and the Government of Ontario is unlikely to be altered by the report of Mr. Justice W.D. Parker who looked into it. The public has already looked into the matter, using its own terms of reference."

24 *Getting Elected*

The provincial election had been called for October 17 and it was essential that I begin to campaign; so I met again with the chiefs of the NDP to choose a riding. Now that I was hooked, their extravagant promises of "any riding I wished" were forgotten and my requests to run against a cabinet minister were brushed aside. They felt that I would probably win any Toronto riding and they urged me to run in the west end where they had no representative, feeling that I might carry two or three neighbouring seats along with me. I flatly refused to run against any sitting Liberal and so High Park, represented by Tory Alf Cowling, was chosen by exclusion. This did not displease me because my medical office of seventeen years was in the centre of the riding.

Mr. Cowling appeared unperturbed: "I'm not surprised—why he was an active Conservative out here for years. I know Morty Shulman well, after all he's a past president of the Parkdale Progressive Conservative Association. The fact that he's running for the NDP—well, he's a millionaire and I don't know how that's going to sit with the socialists." He predicted that I would run a bad third.

The Liberal candidate, Paul Staniszewski, had a similar reaction: "Shulman is an ex-Tory in Socialist clothing. I am in effect running against two Conservatives. This new candidate is not so much interested in the local problems of the riding and the people as he is in promoting himself and pursuing his personal vendetta against the Attorney General."

Government candidates across the province were all unimpressed by my candidacy. Minister of Municipal Affairs Wilf Spooner predicted that I would be soundly defeated; Joe Gould, the PC candidate in Yorkview, said one of the government's great achievements was to dump me into the NDP, and Max Schecter, the government's candidate in Downsview, said that I was not even an issue in the campaign. (I admit to having a feeling of indecent pleasure when all these gentlemen were defeated). The Toronto papers agreed that I had little chance of electoral success. The *Telegram* wrote, "On the basis of the 1963 voting lawyer Paul Staniszewski should take it for the Liberals," and the *Star* said, "When the dust has settled there is a good chance Liberal Paul Staniszewski, who trailed Cowling by 891 votes in the last election, will have the seat."

There was no question in my mind that I would win the election. From the moment of my firing I had received literally thousands of phone calls and letters of support from across the city and I'd carefully kept the names and addresses of all of these well-wishers. When the political campaign began we wrote to these people for their help and most of them volunteered to ring doorbells or to work in the campaign headquarters. The Tories and Liberals were quite literally swamped by an avalanche of manpower and as my volunteers reported back it immediately became obvious that we were going to sweep the riding; in fact there was never a moment of doubt.

As a result of all the publicity the NDP thought I would be an asset in other areas of the province and they began by shipping me to Sudbury. Unfortunately I had never seen that horrible place before and my initial comments to a reporter, comparing the city to the ruins of Hiroshima and the wastes of the Gobi desert did not go over too well with the local residents. The *Sudbury Star* wrote an editorial suggesting that from the rear there was some difficulty in distinguishing me from my horse, and NDP leader MacDonald felt impelled to make a speech saying that I was "mostly wrong" and had missed "the spirit of the people." Sudbury Mayor Grace Hartman suggested that I visit an eye specialist and Premier John Robarts promptly described Sudbury as "delightful, rugged and a community on the move."

After this injudicious beginning I was shipped to Peterborough, where I diplomatically told a union gathering that they would have to show restraints in wages and strikes if the country was to bring inflation under control.

The NDP decided that for the rest of the campaign I should stay in High Park. However, in spite of my help NDPers Eli Martel in Sudbury and Walter Pitman in Peterborough were both elected.

Back in Toronto things went much better. High Park contained a multiracial population of some 40,000, of which 50 per cent were the old Anglo-Saxon residents, 25 per cent were Polish, 15 per cent Ukrainian, 5 per cent Maltese and the remainder a sprinkling of other races. No one was quite sure which way the various groups were leaning but I scored an early victory by winning solid allegiance from the Maltese. This was done over the heads of the leaders of their group, who were solidly Liberal, by writing to Dom Mintoff, head of the Maltese Labour party (and later Prime Minister of that country) and asking for his support. He replied by sending me a letter, which I distributed through the Maltese areas, in which he urged all Maltese to vote for the NDP.

I wasn't the only one with foot-in-mouth disease and the campaign was made easier by the ineptitude of my opponents. The Liberal candidate refused to participate in public question-and-answer meetings and the Conservative Alf Cowling turned off his working-class audience by giving them most unexpected answers. A man at one meeting asked Cowling, "I'm a truck driver and earn $5,000 a year. How can the government pay twice that much for a part-time job as MPP?" The MPP replied that he couldn't live on the $11,000 he received as an MPP. "You must have some other form of income. Everyone has different standards. It's a free country. You can do as you please. You may want to live on $5,000 and I to live on $10,000." Another questioner asked him: "At the present time the working class is taxed up to the neck and work is being taken over by automation. Who will the Tory government tax then?" Mr. Cowling replied "There'll always be someone to tax to keep the ball rolling."

The campaign ended on a bitter note. We had been continually harassed by our election signs being torn down almost as quickly as we could put them up. The office had received several phone tips saying that the signs were being destroyed by Liberal workers and my campaign manager wanted to reciprocate by ripping down their signs. Fortunately I vetoed this and instead hired a detective agency to stake out one of our larger signs. At 2:00 A.M. the day before the election, the detectives watched a young man ripping down the sign and followed him as he put it in his car and took it to a garage behind his home where he placed it along with dozens of others of our signs which had disappeared on previous nights. He turned out to be an executive of the local Tory association.

The election itself was quiet and the results were very one-sided. I had swamped the opposition with 12,888 votes, Staniszewski came second with 6,614 and Cowling had 6,475. I had won every section of the riding and on that exuberant note I began a new career.

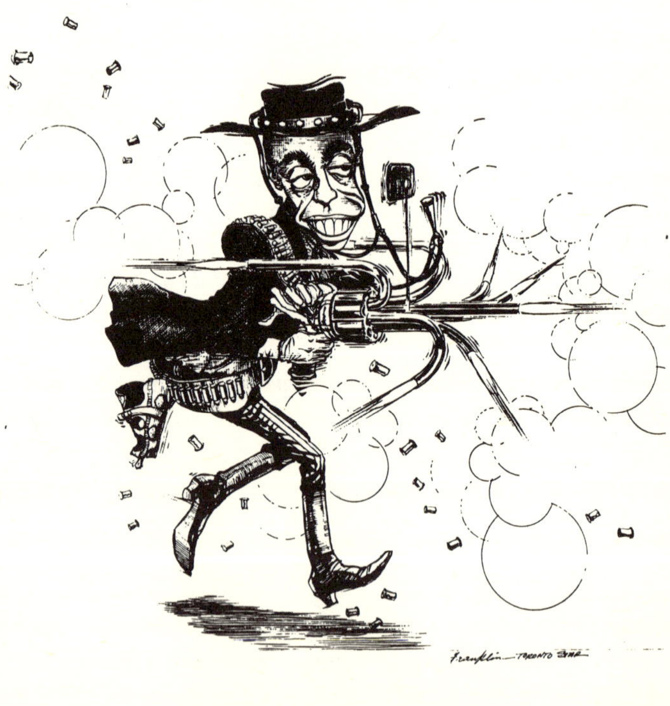